Hormonal and Metabolic Abnormalities in Heart Failure Patients: Pathophysiological Insights and Clinical Relevance

Editor

PASQUALE PERRONE FILARDI

HEART FAILURE CLINICS

www.heartfailure.theclinics.com

Consulting Editor
EDUARDO BOSSONE

Founding Editor
JAGAT NARULA

July 2019 • Volume 15 • Number 3

ELSEVIER

1600 John F. Kennedy Boulevard • Suite 1800 • Philadelphia, Pennsylvania, 19103-2899

http://www.theclinics.com

HEART FAILURE CLINICS Volume 15, Number 3
July 2019 ISSN 1551-7136, ISBN-13: 978-0-323-67799-8

Editor: Stacy Eastman
Developmental Editor: Laura Fisher

Heart Failure Clinics (ISSN 1551-7136) is published quarterly by Elsevier Inc., 360 Park Avenue South, New York, NY 10010-1710. Months of publication are January, April, July, and October. Business and editorial offices: 1600 John F. Kennedy Boulevard, Suite 1800, Philadelphia, PA 19103-2899. Periodicals postage paid at New York, NY, and additional mailing offices. Subscription prices are USD 261.00 per year for US individuals, USD 501.00 per year for US institutions, USD 100.00 per year for US students and residents, USD 300.00 per year for Canadian individuals, USD 580.00 per year for Canadian institutions, USD 315.00 per year for international individuals, USD 580.00 per year for international institutions, and USD 100.00 per year for Canadian and foreign students/residents. To receive student and resident rate, orders must be accompanied by name of affiliated institution, date of term, and the *signature* of program/residency coordinator on institution letterhead. Orders will be billed at individual rate until proof of status is received. Foreign air speed delivery is included in all *Clinics* subscription prices. All prices are subject to change without notice. **POSTMASTER:** Send address changes to *Heart Failure Clinics*, Elsevier Health Sciences Division, Subscription Customer Service, 3251 Riverport Lane, Maryland Heights, MO 63043. **Customer Service: 1-800-654-2452 (US and Canada). From outside of the US and Canada, call 314-447-8871. Fax: 314-447-8029. For print support, E-mail: JournalsCustomerService-usa@elsevier.com. For online support, E-mail: JournalsOnlineSupport-usa@elsevier.com.**

Reprints. For copies of 100 or more of articles in this publication, please contact the Commercial Reprints Department, Elsevier Inc., 360 Park Avenue South, New York, NY 10010-1710. Tel.: 212-633-3874; Fax: 212-633-3820; E-mail: reprints@elsevier.com.

Heart Failure Clinics is covered in *MEDLINE/PubMed (Index Medicus).*

Contributors

CONSULTING EDITOR

EDUARDO BOSSONE, MD, PhD
Division of Cardiology, A. Cardarelli Hospital,
Naples, Italy

EDITOR

PASQUALE PERRONE-FILARDI, MD, PhD
Full Professor of Cardiology, Department
of Advanced Biomedical Sciences,
Federico II University of Naples, Naples,
Italy

AUTHORS

PIERGIUSEPPE AGOSTONI, MD, PhD
Department of "Scompenso Cardiaco e
Cardiologia Clinica," Cardiovascular Section,
Department of Clinical Sciences and
Community Health, University of Milano,
Centro Cardiologico Monzino, IRCCS, Milan,
Italy

ANTONIO AMBROSIO, MD
Department of Advanced Biomedical
Sciences, Section of Cardiology, Federico II
University of Naples, Naples, Italy

MICHELE ARCOPINTO, MD
Department of Translational Medical Sciences,
Federico II University of Naples, Naples, Italy;
Emergency Department, Cardarelli Hospital,
Naples, Italy

RAGAVENDRA R. BALIGA, MD, PhD
Division of Cardiovascular Medicine, The Ohio
State University Wexner Medical Center, Davis
Heart and Lung Research Institute, Columbus,
Ohio, USA

LUCA BARDI, MD
Department of Advanced Biomedical
Sciences, Section of Cardiology, Federico II
University of Naples, Naples, Italy

LEONARDO BENCIVENGA, MD
Graduate Medical Fellow, Department of
Translational Medical Sciences, Division of
Geriatrics, Federico II University of Naples,
Naples, Italy

BERNADETTE BIONDI, MD
Professor of Internal Medicine, Department of
Clinical Medicine and Surgery, Federico II
University of Naples, Naples, Italy

EDUARDO BOSSONE, MD, PhD
Division of Cardiology, A. Cardarelli Hospital,
Naples, Italy

ANTONIO CITTADINI, MD
Department of Translational Medical Sciences,
Federico II University of Naples,
Interdisciplinary Research Centre in
Biomedical Materials, Naples, Italy

ANNAMARIA COLAO, MD, PhD
Dipartimento di Medicina Clinica e Chirurgia,
Sezione di Endocrinologia, Federico II
University of Naples, Naples, Italy

CRISTINA CONTIELLO, MS
Department of Advanced Biomedical
Sciences, Section of Cardiology, Federico II
University of Naples, Naples, Italy

ROBERTA D'ASSANTE, PhD
Istituto di Ricovero e Cura a Carattere
Scientifico SDN, Naples, Italy

FABIANA DE MARTINO, MD
Department of "Scompenso Cardiaco e
Cardiologia Clinica," Centro Cardiologico
Monzino, IRCCS, Milano, Italy;
Department of Advanced Biomedical
Sciences, Section of Cardiology, Federico II
University of Naples, Naples, Italy

ANNA MARIA DE ROBERTO, MD
Department of Advanced Biomedical
Sciences, Section of Cardiology, Federico II
University of Naples, Naples, Italy

SIMONA DELL'AVERSANA, MD
Department of Advanced Biomedical
Sciences, Section of Cardiology, Federico II
University of Naples, Naples, Italy

SANTO DELLEGROTTAGLIE, MD, PhD
Division of Cardiology, Ospedale Accreditato
Villa dei Fiori, Acerra, Naples, Italy; Zena and
Michael A. Wiener Cardiovascular Institute/
Marie-Josee and Henry R. Kravis Center for
Cardiovascular Health, Icahn School of
Medicine at Mount Sinai, New York, New York,
USA

PABLO DEMELO-RODRIGUEZ, MD, PhD
Venous Thromboembolism Unit, Internal
Medicine Department, Hospital General
Universitario Gregorio Marañón, School of
Medicine, Universidad Complutense de
Madrid, Madrid, Spain

PIERFRANCESCO DI NAPOLI, MD
Department of Advanced Biomedical
Sciences, Section of Cardiology, Federico II
University of Naples, Naples, Italy

CAROLINA DI SOMMA, MD, PhD
Istituto di Ricovero e Cura a
Carattere Scientifico SDN, Naples,
Italy

GAETANO DIANA, MD
Department of Advanced Biomedical
Sciences, Section of Cardiology,
Federico II University of Naples, Naples,
Italy

IMMACOLATA ESPOSITO, MD
Department of Advanced Biomedical
Sciences, Section of Cardiology, Federico II
University of Naples, Naples, Italy

LUCA ESPOSITO, MD
Department of Advanced Biomedical
Sciences, Section of Cardiology, Federico II
University of Naples, Naples, Italy

FRANCESCA FERRAZZANO, MD
Department of Advanced Biomedical
Sciences, Section of Cardiology, Federico II
University of Naples, Naples, Italy

PAOLA GARGIULO, MD, PhD
IRCCS SDN, Naples, Italy

LUDOVICA F.S. GRASSO, MD
Dipartimento di Medicina Clinica e Chirurgia,
Sezione di Endocrinologia, Federico II
University of Naples, Naples, Italy

MONICA IANNIRUBERTO, MS
Department of Advanced Biomedical
Sciences, Section of Cardiology, Federico II
University of Naples, Naples, Italy

LUCIA LA MURA, MD
Department of Advanced Biomedical
Sciences, Section of Cardiology, Federico II
University of Naples, Naples, Italy

MARK LANDER, MBBS, MRCP
Department of Acute Medicine, University
College London Hospitals NHS Foundation
Trust, London, United Kingdom

DARIO LEOSCO, MD, PhD
Associate Professor, Department of
Translational Medical Sciences, Division of
Geriatrics, Federico II University of Naples,
Naples, Italy

DANIELA LICCARDO, PhD
Research Post-Doctoral Fellow, Department of
Translational Medical Sciences, Division of
Geriatrics, Federico II University of Naples,
Naples, Italy

DAMIANO MAGRÌ, MD, PhD
Department of Clinical and Molecular
Medicine, Azienda Ospedaliera Sant'Andrea,
"Sapienza" Università degli Studi di Roma,
Roma, Italy

ALBERTO M. MARRA, MD
Istituto di Ricovero e Cura a Carattere
Scientifico SDN, Naples, Italy

FABIO MARSICO, MD, PhD
Department of Advanced Biomedical
Sciences, Section of Cardiology, Federico II
University of Naples, Naples, Italy; Center for
Congenital Heart Disease, University Hospital
Inselspital, University of Bern, Bern,
Switzerland

ROSA MENNELLA, MS
Department of Advanced Biomedical
Sciences, Section of Cardiology, Federico II
University of Naples, Naples, Italy

FEDERICA MOSCUCCI, MD
Dipartimento di Scienze Cardiovascolari,
Respiratorie, Nefrologiche, Anestesiologiche e
Geriatriche, "Sapienza" Università degli Studi
di Roma, Roma, Italy

CARMEN NAPOLITANO, MD
Graduate Medical Fellow, Department of
Translational Medical Sciences, Division of
Geriatrics, Federico II University of Naples,
Naples, Italy

ROBERTA PAOLILLO
PhD Student, Department of Advanced
Biomedical Sciences, Section of Cardiology,
Federico II University of Naples, Naples,
Italy

STEFANIA PAOLILLO, MD, PhD
Department of Advanced Biomedical
Sciences, Federico II University of Naples,
Mediterranean Clinic, Istituto di Ricovero e
Cura a Carattere Scientifico SDN, Naples, Italy

ANTONIO PARENTE, MD
Department of Advanced Biomedical
Sciences, Federico II University of Naples,
Naples, Italy

CARMINE EMANUELE PASCALE, RT
Division of Cardiology, Ospedale Accreditato
Villa dei Fiori, Acerra, Naples, Italy

PASQUALE PERRONE-FILARDI, MD, PhD
Full Professor of Cardiology, Department
of Advanced Biomedical Sciences,
Federico II University of Naples, Naples,
Italy

ROSARIO PIVONELLO, MD, PhD
Dipartimento di Medicina Clinica e Chirurgia,
Sezione di Endocrinologia, Federico II
University of Naples, Naples, Italy

MARIA PRASTARO, MD
Department of Advanced Biomedical
Sciences, Section of Cardiology,
Federico II University of Naples, Naples,
Italy

FRANCESCO RENGA, MD
Department of Advanced Biomedical
Sciences, Section of Cardiology,
Federico II University of Naples, Naples,
Italy

GIUSEPPE RENGO, MD, PhD
Associate Professor, Department of
Translational Medical Sciences, Division
of Geriatrics, Federico II University of
Naples, Naples, Italy; Istituti Clinici
Scientifici Maugeri SpA Società
Benefit (ICS Maugeri SpA SB),
Telese Terme, Italy

ANDREA SALZANO, MD, MRCP
Department of Cardiovascular Sciences,
NIHR Leicester Biomedical Research
Centre, University of Leicester, Glenfield
Hospital, Leicester, United Kingdom;
Department of Translational Medical
Sciences, Federico II University of Naples,
Naples, Italy

ALESSANDRA SCATTEIA, MD
Division of Cardiology, Ospedale Accreditato
Villa dei Fiori, Acerra, Naples, Italy

ALESSANDRA SCHIAVO, MD
Department of Translational Medical Sciences,
Federico II University of Naples, Naples,
Italy

SUSANNA SCIOMER, MD
Dipartimento di Scienze Cardiovascolari,
Respiratorie, Nefrologiche, Anestesiologiche e
Geriatriche, "Sapienza" Università degli Studi
di Roma, Roma, Italy

TORU SUZUKI, MD, PhD, FRCP
Department of Cardiovascular Sciences, NIHR
Leicester Biomedical Research Centre,
University of Leicester, Glenfield Hospital,
Leicester, United Kingdom

LUCIA VISAGGI, MD
Graduate Medical Fellow, Department of
Translational Medical Sciences, Division of
Geriatrics, Federico II University of Naples,
Naples, Italy

MARIA CRISTINA VOZZELLA, MD
Department of Advanced Biomedical
Sciences, Section of Cardiology,
Federico II University of Naples, Naples,
Italy

Contents

Heart failure is a clinical syndrome characterized by left ventricular dysfunction and/or elevated intracardiac pressures, with a prevalence of about 1% to 2% in the general population. In the last decades, many metabolic disorders have been studied as linked with heart failure. Diabetes mellitus and insulin resistance are strictly related to heart failure, with a bidirectional link, where each can influence the other. The aim of this article is to report the role of glucose metabolism abnormalities in the development of heart failure, defining the epidemiology and assessing pathophysiology and prognosis of heart failure related to glucose metabolism disorders.

A strict bidirectional relationship exists between diabetes mellitus and heart failure. Diabetic cardiomyopathy is a specific cardiac manifestation of patients with diabetes characterized by left ventricular hypertrophy and diastolic dysfunction in the early phase up to overt heart failure with reduced systolic function in the advanced stages. The pathogenesis of this condition is multifactorial and recognizes as main promoting factors the presence of insulin resistance and hyperglycemia. Diabetic cardiomyopathy exerts a negative prognostic impact in affected patients and no target treatments are currently available. More efforts are needed to better define the diagnostic and therapeutic approach in this specific setting.

The interplay between metabolic syndrome (MetS) and heart failure (HF) is intricate. Population studies show that MetS confers an increased risk to develop HF and this effect is mediated by insulin resistance (IR). However, obesity, a key component in MetS and common partner of IR, is protective in patients with established HF, although IR confers an increased risk of dying by HF. Such phenomenon, known as "obesity paradox," accounts for the complexity of the HF-MetS relationship. Because IR impacts more on outcomes than MetS itself, the former may be considered the actual target for MetS in HF patients.

Anemia and iron deficiency (ID) represent 2 prevalent, often interrelated, comorbidities in heart failure (HF). Both of them are significantly related to functional capacity and are undoubted predictors of poor prognosis in patients with HF. Although anemia and ID both have "global" detrimental effects, these 2 conditions are too often overlooked in cardiology daily clinical practice. The present review sought to summarize briefly the prevalence and the underlying pathophysiologic mechanisms of anemia and ID as regards HF severity (ie, exercise capacity) and prognosis.

The model used to explain the pathophysiologic substrate and progressive worsening in chronic heart failure (CHF) is based on the hyperactivity of renin-angiotensin-aldosterone system and adrenergic pathway. Although the neurohormonal medical approach has many advantages, it has several pitfalls, as demonstrated by high rates of CHF mortality and hospitalization. A growing body of evidence has led to the hypothesis that CHF is a multiple hormone deficiency syndrome, characterized by a reduced anabolic drive that has relevant functional and prognostic implications. The aim of this review is to summarize the evidence of reduced drive of main anabolic axes in CHF.

A growing body of evidence led to the hypothesis that heart failure (HF) could be considered a multiple hormone deficiency syndrome. Deficiencies in the main anabolic axes cannot be considered as mere epiphenomena, are very common in HF, and are clearly associated with poor cardiovascular performance and outcomes. Growth hormone deficiency and testosterone deficiency play a pivotal role and the replacement treatment is an innovative therapy that should be considered. This article appraises the current evidence regarding growth hormone and testosterone deficiencies in HF and reviews novel findings about the treatment of these conditions in HF.

The cardiovascular system is one of the main targets of thyroid hormone action, and triiodothyronine deficiency has crucial consequences on cardiac structure and function. Patients with overt or subclinical hypothyroidism should be treated with levothyroxine to improve their cardiovascular function and the potential risk of heart failure. Even patients with thyroid hormone deficiency and heart failure should receive replacement doses of levothyroxine to improve their prognosis and worsening of the cardiovascular function. An innovative therapeutic multifactorial approach could improve the progression of heart failure. There is a potential beneficial effect of thyroid hormones and their analogs in patients with heart failure.

In patients with acromegaly, chronic GH and IGF-I excess commonly causes a specific cardiomyopathy characterized by a concentric cardiac hypertrophy associated with diastolic dysfunction and, in later stages, with systolic dysfunction ending in heart failure in untreated and uncontrolled patients. Additional relevant cardiovascular complications are represented by arterial hypertension, valvulopathies, arrhythmias, and vascular endothelial dysfunction, which, together with the respiratory and metabolic complications, contribute to the development of cardiac disease and the increase cardiovascular risk in acromegaly. Disease duration plays a pivotal role in the determination of acromegalic cardiomyopathy. The main functional disturbance in acromegalic cardiomyopathy is the diastolic dysfunction, observed in 11% to 58% of patients, it is usually mild, without clinical consequence, and the progression to systolic dysfunction is generally uncommon, not seen or observed in less than 3% of the patients. Consequently, the presence of overt CHF is rare in acromegaly, ranging between 1 and 4%, in patients with untreated and uncontrolled disease. Control of acromegaly, induced by either pituitary surgery or medical therapy improves cardiac structure and performance, limiting the progression of acromegaly cardiomyopathy to CHF. However, when CHF is associated with dilative cardiomyopathy, it is generally not reversible, despite the treatment of the acromegaly.

Despite improvements in management and therapeutic approach in the last decades, heart failure is still associated with high mortality rates. The sustained enhancement in the sympathetic nervous system tone, observed in patients with heart failure, causes alteration in β-adrenergic receptor signaling and function. This latter phenomenon is the result of several heart failure–related molecular abnormalities involving adrenergic receptors, G-protein–coupled receptor kinases, and β-arrestins. This article summarizes novel encouraging preclinical strategies to reactivate β-adrenergic receptor signaling in heart failure, including pharmacologic and gene therapy approaches, and attempts to translate acquired notions into the clinical setting.

Alterations in myocardial energy metabolism as demonstrated by magnetic resonance spectroscopy (MRS) are critically involved in heart failure development. ^{1}H-MRS allows investigation of the role of myocardial lipid accumulation in the pathophysiology of heart failure. With ^{31}P-MRS, the most useful parameter is the cardiac adenosine triphosphate to phosphocreatine ratio, which is typically reduced in the failing heart and correlates with cardiac functional status. Currently, MRS is mostly limited to the research setting, but recent technical and methodological developments might substantially improve its clinical applicability for initial characterization and successive monitoring of patients with heart failure.

HEART FAILURE CLINICS

SERIES OF RELATED INTEREST

Cardiology Clinics
http://www.cardiology.theclinics.com/

THE CLINICS ARE AVAILABLE ONLINE!
Access your subscription at:
www.theclinics.com

Preface

Understanding the Pathophysiology to Improve the Therapeutic Management: Focus on Metabolic and Hormonal Comorbidities in Heart Failure

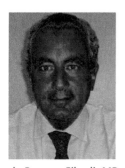
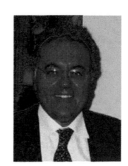

Pasquale Perrone Filardi, MD, PhD   Eduardo Bossone, MD, PhD, FCCP, FESC, FACC

Editors

Heart failure (HF) is a leading cause of mortality and morbidity worldwide.[1]. Despite remarkable progress in the therapeutic management of HF, poor survival and high readmission rates are still observed.[2] The presence of multiple comorbidities and, in particular, of metabolic and hormonal disorders, complicates the diagnostic and therapeutic management of HF patients and is responsible for a progression of the disease. Diabetes mellitus and insulin resistance are highly prevalent in HF patients and responsible for poor prognosis and for a typical HF phenotype.[3] Moreover, a growing body of evidence led to the hypothesis that HF could be considered a multiple hormone deficiency syndrome, concluding that the observed deficiencies in the main anabolic axes cannot be considered simple epiphenomena, exhibiting a clear association with poor cardiovascular performance and outcomes.[4] In the present issue, we aimed to focus the attention on the main metabolic and hormonal comorbidities observed in HF patients, in terms of their pathophysiological impact on the baseline cardiac condition, of their specific clinical relevance in this setting, and of possible therapeutic approaches. In the last few years, new therapeutic approaches to metabolic and hormonal disorders have demonstrated a positive impact on quality of life, cardiac function,

mortality, and HF progression, opening new scenarios in the therapeutic approach to HF. We hope that the contents of this issue could stimulate the interest of the scientific community on this specific topic, aiming for an implementation of research studies and working together to further improve HF patients' quality of life and long-term prognosis.

Let us thank Dr Stefania Paolillo and Dr Paola Gargiulo for support in the editing process.

Enjoy the reading,.

Pasquale Perrone Filardi, MD, PhD
Department of Advanced
Biomedical Sciences
Federico II University of Naples
Via Pansini, 5
Naples 80131, Italy

Eduardo Bossone, MD, PhD, FCCP, FESC, FACC
Division of Cardiology
Cardarelli Hospital
Via A. Cardarelli, 9
Naples 80131, Italy

E-mail addresses:
fpperron@unina.it (P. Perrone Filardi)
ebossone@hotmail.com (E. Bossone)

Heart Failure Clin 15 (2019) xi–xii
https://doi.org/10.1016/j.hfc.2019.04.001
1551-7136/19/© 2019 Published by Elsevier Inc.

REFERENCES

1. Braunwald E. Heart failure. JACC Heart Fail 2013;1: 1–20.
2. Laribi S, Aouba A, Nikolaou M, et al. Trends in death attributed to heart failure over the past two decades in Europe. Eur J Heart Fail 2012;14(3):234–9.
3. Seferovic PM, Petrie MC, Filippatos GS, et al. Type 2 diabetes mellitus and heart failure: a position statement from the Heart Failure Association of the European Society of Cardiology. Eur J Heart Fail 2018;20(5):853–72.
4. Arcopinto M, Salzano A, Bossone E, et al. Multiple hormone deficiencies in chronic heart failure. Int J Cardiol 2015;184:421–3.

Glucose Metabolism Abnormalities in Heart Failure Patients
Insights and Prognostic Relevance

Fabio Marsico, MD, PhD[a,b,*], Paola Gargiulo, MD, PhD[c],
Alberto M. Marra, MD[c], Antonio Parente, MD[a],
Stefania Paolillo, MD, PhD[a,d]

KEYWORDS

- Heart failure • Glucose metabolism abnormalities • Diabetes mellitus • Insulin resistance
- Hyperglycemia • Insulin sensitivity

KEY POINTS

- Heart failure is a clinical syndrome characterized by left ventricular dysfunction and/or elevated intracardiac pressures, with a prevalence of about 1% to 2% in the general population.
- There are several factors involved in heart failure development, from ischemic heart disease to metabolic disorders, passing through genetic etiology.
- Insulin resistance is a frequent finding among heart failure patients, with a bidirectional link between them.
- The homeostasis model assessment index has proved to be a robust and reliable tool for the assessment of insulin resistance.
- Heart failure can be considered the major cause of hospitalization in patients with glucose metabolism abnormalities.

INTRODUCTION

Heart failure (HF) is a clinical syndrome caused by structural and/or functional cardiac abnormality, resulting in a reduced left ventricular function, and/or elevated intracardiac pressures.[1] The prevalence of HF is approximately 1% to 2% of the adult population, rising to at least 10% over 70 years of age.[1–5] Nowadays it is not possible to define a precise etiology of HF, but there are several factors involved in HF development, from ischemic heart disease to metabolic disorders, passing through genetic etiology.[1] Focusing on metabolic disorders responsible of HF development, there is a wide spectrum of metabolic abnormalities that can lead to HF.

In the last years, an increase of prevalence in many metabolic disorders has been observed, in particular in the glucose metabolism abnormalities rate,[6] in the context of westernized lifestyles, high-fat diets, and decreased exercise, leading to increasing levels of obesity, insulin resistance (IR), compensatory hyperinsulinemia, and ultimately, type 2 diabetes mellitus (T2DM).[6] Although

Disclosure: The authors have nothing to disclose.
Funding: Dr F. Marsico has been supported by a research grant provided by the Cardiovascular Pathophysiology and Therapeutics PhD program.
[a] Department of Advanced Biomedical Sciences, Federico II University, Via Pansini 5, Naples 80131, Italy;
[b] Center for Congenital Heart Disease, University Hospital Inselspital, University of Bern, Switzerland;
[c] IRCCS SDN, Via Gianturco, 113, Naples 80142, Italy; [d] Mediterranean Clinic, Via Orazio 2, Naples 80122, Italy
* Corresponding author. Via Pansini, 5, Naples I-80131, Italy.
E-mail address: fabiomarsico84@gmail.com

the most known cardiac (not ischemic) nosologic entity related to glucose metabolism disorders is diabetic cardiomyopathy, IR, regardless of association with T2DM, is a frequent finding among HF patients, with a prevalence ranging from 33% to 70%.[7–9] There is a bidirectional link between IR and HF, where although IR can predict HF, it often develops in HF patients, with more severe symptoms and worse clinical outcomes.[10–13] The degree of IR is significantly related with worsened clinical presentation and a poor prognosis in patients with HF, and it is known that metformin can prevent HF progression, improving exercise capacity.[7,10,12–14]

The scope of this appraisal is to report the role of glucose metabolism abnormalities in the development of HF, defining a classification and diagnosis of glucose metabolism defects, which can lead to T2DM, and assessing pathophysiology and prognosis of HF related to glucose metabolism abnormalities.

CLASSIFICATION OF GLUCOSE METABOLISM ABNORMALITIES

Glucose metabolism disorders are a wide spectrum of abnormalities, characterized by elevated levels of blood glucose and impaired levels of circulating insulin. The actual classification of glucose metabolism abnormalities is based on recommendations from the World Health Organization (WHO) and the American Diabetes Association (ADA)[6,15–17] (Box 1).

Box 1
Different types of glucose metabolism disorders

Type 1 diabetes mellitus

Type 2 diabetes mellitus

Other specific types of diabetes mellitus

    Genetic mutation forms

    Secondary to other diseases

        Diseases of the exocrine pancreas

        Endocrinopathies

    Drug or chemically induced

    Infective forms

Gestational diabetes mellitus

Prediabetic disorders

    Impaired fasting glucose

    Impaired glucose tolerance

    Insulin resistance

There are classic 4 main etiologic categories of DM (see **Box 1**) identified as

Type 1 DM (caused by destruction of pancreatic beta-cells, progressing to absolute insulin deficiency; although is typical of young age, it can occur at any age)

T2DM (characterized by a combination of IR and beta-cells failure)

gestational DM

Other specific types of DM (this entity includes single genetic mutation forms, DM secondary to other diseases, drug- or chemically induced DM, and infective forms)

Beyond these categories is group of entities called prediabetic disorders that are strictly related to cardiovascular (CV) events and in particular to HF development, and that includes a variety of disorders to be discussed.[6,17]

Different Types of Prediabetic Disorders

All the types of glucose metabolism disorders (see **Box 1**) can often be considered as precursors of blown DM (generally T2DM), but in many cases are isolated and not related to the presence of T2DM. Between these entities, there are impaired fasting glucose (IFG) and impaired glucose tolerance (IGT), that are often referred to as prediabetes, reflecting the natural history of progression from normoglycemia to T2DM.[6] Considered the normal oscillation of fasting plasma glucose values day by day, many times these forms of glucose metabolism abnormalities could pass misdiagnosed. For this reason, IFG and IGT often can only be recognized by the results of an oral glucose tolerance test (OGTT).[6] However, the most important form of glucose metabolism disorders, that, although could lead to T2DM, is common also in nondiabetic patients, is IR. The concept of IR was proposed first time in 1936, and is generally defined as reduced biological action of insulin, such as inhibition of hepatic glucose production and insulin-mediated glucose disposal.[18–20] There is a known correlation between obesity and IR development. In particular, patients with IR who are not obese by traditional weight criteria may have an increased percentage of body fat distributed predominantly in the abdominal region.[17] This type of glucose metabolism abnormality frequently goes undiagnosed for many years, because in the beginning there is not a clear hyperglycemia, which develops gradually, without showing the classic symptoms of diabetes.[17] Nevertheless, many patients experience CV events, including also the developing of HF, explaining the role of IR in HF pathogenesis also in nondiabetic patients.[17] As result of normal or elevated levels of insulin in patients with IR, the higher blood glucose levels cannot be compensated for by high levels of circulating insulin, because of the low effect of insulin. Thus, insulin secretion is defective in a first step in these patients and insufficient to compensate for IR. In a second step, considering the possible development of T2DM, also levels of circulating insulin become insufficient, requiring a supplement of them.[17]

DIAGNOSIS OF GLUCOSE METABOLISM ABNORMALITIES
Diabetes Mellitus, Impaired Fasting Glucose, and Impaired Glucose Tolerance

As general rule, DM is defined by an elevated level of blood glucose. Based on this assumption, the World Health Organization (WHO) criteria for diagnosis of glucose metabolism abnormalities are based on fasting plasma glucose (FPG) and 2-hour postload plasma glucose (2hPG) (when there is not an overt hyperglycemia [OGTT]) concentration[6,21] (**Box 2**). On the other hand, in addition to these parameters of glucose metabolism disorders diagnosis, the ADA recommends use of glycated hemoglobin A_{1C} (HbA$_{1C}$). Therefore, for the diagnosis of DM, IFG, and IGT, there are several parameters to use, different between WHO and ADA. In particular, for WHO, the cut-points are the following[6]:

1. Diabetes mellitus
   - HbA$_{1C}$ can be used, with a cut-point of at least 6.5%

Box 2
Diagnostic evaluation of glucose metabolism disorders (according to the World Health Organization and the American Diabetes Association)

Diabetes mellitus

   Glycated hemoglobin A_{1C} (HbA$_{1C}$)

   Fasting plasma glucose

   2-h postload plasma glucose (OGTT)

Impaired glucose tolerance

   Fasting plasma glucose

   2-h postload plasma glucose (OGTT)

Impaired fasting glucose

   Fasting plasma glucose

Insulin resistance

   HOMA index

- FPG is recommended, with a cut-point of at least 126 mg/dL
- 2hPG is recommended, with a cut-point of at least 200 mg/dL
2. Impaired glucose tolerance
   - FPG is recommended, with a cut-point less than 126 mg/d
   - 2hPG is recommended, with a cut-point of at least140 but less than 200 mg/dL
3. Impaired fasting glucose: FPG is recommended, with a cut-point of 110 to 125 mg/dL

Regarding ADA, the cut-points are the following[6]:

1. Diabetes mellitus
   - HbA$_{1C}$ is recommended, with a cut-point of at least 6,5%
   - FPG is recommended, with a cut-point of at least 126 mg/dL
   - 2hPG is recommended, with a cut-point of at least 200 mg/dL
2. Impaired glucose tolerance: FPG is recommended, with a cut-point of less than 126 mg/dL
3. Impaired fasting glucose: FPG is recommended, with a cut-point of 110 to 125 mg/dL

Insulin Resistance

Regarding IR, the homeostasis model assessment (HOMA) index has proved to be a robust and reliable tool for the assessment of IR (see **Box 2**). This method is based on a homeostatic mathematic model considering FPG and fasting plasma insulin. In particular, HOMA-IR is calculated using the formula (fasting glucose [mmol/L] $\times$ fasting insulin [mIU/L]/22.5). Several studies[18,20,22–28] have assessed a normal range value for HOMA index that is considered now between 0,23 and 2,5.

Strategy for Early Detection of Impaired Glucose Metabolism

As known, DM does not cause specific symptoms for many years, which could explain the great number of T2DM cases undiagnosed over several years. Overall, this could be the reason of several CV disorders related to DM that occur before the diagnosis of DM. On the other hand, as known, IR (a frequent precursor of T2DM) is always asymptomatic and is not associated with hyperglycemia. For this reason, it is more difficult to detect with routine examinations.[6] However, screening of hyperglycemia (or of IR), should be targeted to high-risk individuals with CV disease and HF.[6] So, according to current guidelines,[6] the approaches for early detection of glucose metabolism abnormalities are

- Measuring PG or HbA_{1C}
- Using demographic and clinical characteristics to determine the likelihood of impaired glucose metabolism (for the eventual evaluation of HOMA-index)
- Evaluation of the presence of possible risk factors of glucose metabolism disorders, CV events, and HF (for the eventual evaluation of HOMA-index)

PATHOPHYSIOLOGICAL INSIGHTS OF HEART FAILURE RELATED TO GLUCOSE METABOLISM DISORDERS

As previously described, IR is a direct precursor of T2DM, and the consequent compensatory hyperinsulinemia peculiar of IR, with consequent elevated levels of PG, associated with clustering of CV risk, can lead to several CV diseases.[6] As known, T2DM patients are generally obese (or with higher levels of fat abdominally distributed), and the release of free fatty acid (FFA) from adipose

tissue directly impairs insulin sensitivity[6,29] (**Fig. 1**). So, the primum movens is IR, with several consequent mechanisms involved in HF presentation and progression. However, well known is the bidirectional link between IR and HF.[11] Several studies have indicated that DM and IR are not only causative factors of HF,[30–32] but patients with HF and DM or IR show a more aggressive form of left ventricular dysfunction, with higher mortality rates.[33] IR is the entity with higher prevalence in HF patients (up to 60%),[34] with a complex pathophysiological interaction, since IR may be the cause and consequence of HF at the same time.[30] Similarly, DM has a prevalence of 10% to 40% in patients with HF,[35] showing a high prevalence, but lower than IR. This could explain the more important and potential role of IR in HF development (and vice versa), compared with DM, that was widely discussed in the last years.[8,9,30]

Pathophysiology of Heart Failure in Insulin Resistance and Diabetes Mellitus

Well known is the role of IR and DM in several functional, metabolic, and structural alterations that

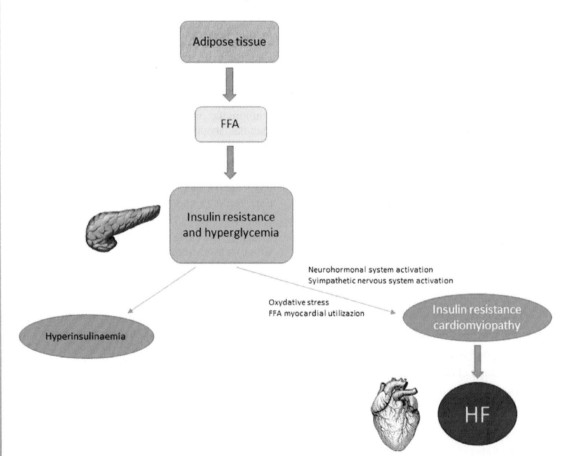

Fig. 1. Pathophysiology of HF development related to insulin resistance.

involve myocardial tissue and can lead to HF (see **Fig. 1**). In the initial stage of HF, there is a change in substrate utilization, where glucose becomes the primary substrate oxidized.[9] Hyperglycemia is responsible for several cellular pathway abnormalities, going from increased polyol, modification of proteins, and formation of advanced glycation end products, to increased protein kinase C expression, a phenomenon leading to overproduction of superoxide and consequent oxidative stress[30,36] (see **Fig. 1**). On the other hand, the increase of FFA myocardial uptake, typical of diabetes and obesity, leads to long-chain FFA oxidation and to a disproportionate oxidative request to mitochondria with uncoupling of mitochondrial oxidative phosphorylation[30,37] (see **Fig. 1**). In addition, the impaired expression of contractile proteins is responsible for depressed myofibrillar ATP activities and abnormalities of the sarcoplasmic reticular and sarcolemma calcium transport process, with consequent calcium overload and impaired diastolic function.[30,38]

Hyperactivation of Adrenergic System

Another consideration is on the impairment of cardiac sympathetic innervation, commonly observed in HF patients affected by DM and/or IR. In a recent study, Paolillo and colleagues[34] showed in HF patients without DM, but with IR, a more impaired cardiac sympathetic innervation compared with non-IR patients, indicating a chronic adrenergic hyperactivity that correlates with high levels of insulinemia and with HOMA index. In the same year, Rengo and colleagues[39] reported that levels of GRK2, a protein kinase involved in the desensitization of cardiac beta-receptors, are significantly more elevated in HF patients with DM compared with nondiabetic patients with HF, meaning a stronger adrenergic activation, known to be involved in progression and worsening of HF.

EPIDEMIOLOGY OF HEART FAILURE IN GLUCOSE METABOLISM ABNORMALITIES AND VICE VERSA

The bidirectional link between HF and glucose metabolism disorders has been discussed. Well known is the prevalence of HF in the general population, about 1% to 2%,[1–5] rising to 12% to 30% in diabetic patients.[40,41] Glucose metabolism abnormalities (in particular DM and IR) are independent risk factors for the development of HF. In the Framingham study, the relative risk of HF in patients with T2DM was doubled for men and 6 times as high in women.[6,42] These data were confirmed by the National Health and Nutrition Examination

Survey, where T2DM was showed to be an independent predictor of HF (HR 1.85, 95% confidence interval [CI] 1.51–2.28).[43]

On the other hand, the prevalence of DM in the general population is about 6% to 8%,[6] but rises to 12% to 30% in HF patients, as described by MacDonald and colleagues.[44] However, HF patients are older than the general population. This could be considered a selection bias. The role of glucose metabolism disorders in development of HF and the major prevalence of glucose metabolism abnormalities (in particular DM and IR, as previously described) in HF patients are widely known. Confirming these data, the TOSCA registry,[7] a recent Italian registry made of 526 patients (81% male, age 62.5 $\pm$ 12.2 years) has shown a prevalence of IR in HF patients of 30% to 35%, in line with previous studies, demonstrating the great impact of glucose metabolism abnormalities on HF.

PROGNOSIS OF HEART FAILURE RELATED TO GLUCOSE METABOLISM ABNORMALITIES
Great Trials

HF can be considered the major cause of hospitalization in patients with glucose metabolism abnormalities. These data have been confirmed by the Hypertension, Microalbuminuria or Proteinuria, Cardiovascular Events and Ramipril (DIABHYCAR) trial,[45] with a mortality 12-fold higher in patients with HF and glucose metabolism disorders, compared with patients without HF (36% vs 3%). On the other hand, in the BEta blocker STroke (BEST) trial, impaired glucose metabolism increased the risk of hospitalization in HF patients, with T2DM as independent predictor of mortality, mostly for HF.[46] More recently, the Metoprolol CR/XL Randomized Intervention Trial in Congestive Heart Failure (MERIT-HF),[47] showed HF patients with glucose metabolism alterations to be more hospitalized than patients free from DM.

Previous Studies

A previous study of Suskin and colleagues[12] examined 663 patients with abnormalities in glucose metabolism (DM or IR) and HF, assessing prognostic role of glucose metabolism, in particular, evaluating functional class, 6-minute walking performance, and left ventricular function. In this cohort of patients, they found a greater proportion of diabetic patients compared with nondiabetic patients in New York Heart Association (NYHA) class III/IV (161 vs 77, $P=.011$), with a higher value of insulin in nondiabetic patients in NYHA class III/IV compared with NYHA class I/II (19.6 $\pm$ 2.3 vs 10.2 $\pm$ 0.6 mU, $P<.005$). In addition, among nondiabetic patients, significantly more NYHA class III/IV patients had elevated HOMA-index levels (44% vs 28%, $P<.005$) compared with NYHA class I/II patients. These data were confirmed also for the 6-minute walking distance, which was significantly shorter in diabetic patients compared with nondiabetic patients (369 ± 7 vs 385 ± 4 m, $P=.03$). Furthermore, patients with impaired HOMA-index had a significantly shorter 6-minute walking distance than those with normal values (372 ± 7 vs 391 ± 5 m, $P=.02$).

A more recent study of Doehner and colleagues[13] evaluated insulin sensitivity in 105 male patients with HF. After a mean follow up of 44 ± 4 months, patients with an insulin sensitivity below the median value had a worse survival (61% at 2 years) compared with patients with an insulin sensitivity above the median value (83% at 2 years) (relative risk [RR] 0.38, 95% CI 0.21–0.67, $P = .001$). Furthermore, insulin sensitivity resulted independent predictor of mortality in the study cohort.

Therapeutic Possibilities

Considering the impact on prognosis of glucose metabolism abnormalities, it is possible affirm that DM and IR can be considered as potential target of HF. Although the role of several new pharmacologic agents in the reduction of mortality in HF diabetic patients is known,[48] little is known about the potential treatment of IR and its impact on HF prognosis. Considering this assumption, Wong and colleagues[14] randomized in a double-blind, placebo-controlled study 62 nondiabetic HF patients to receive either 4 months of metformin or matching placebo. Compared with placebo, metformin decreased HOMA-index, improving also the secondary endpoint of the slope of the ratio of minute ventilation to carbon dioxide production (VE/VCO$_2$ slope). These data confirm the hypothesis that treatment of IR should be protective in patients with HF.

Interesting data for the prevention of HF in patients with DM come from the results of clinical studies with sodium-glucose cotransporter 2 (SGLT2) inhibitors. In particular, the EMPA-REG OUTCOME trial[49] demonstrated that treatment with empagliflozin reduced hospitalization for HF in diabetic patients at high CV risk and that this effect was independent from the presence of HF at baseline.

On the other hand, there are several ongoing trials[50] evaluating the efficacy of SGLT2 in patients with HFpEF (EMPEROR-preserved) and in patients with HFrEF (EMPEROR-reduced), including HF patients without DM with the composite primary endpoint of time to first event of adjudicated CV death or adjudicated HF.

SUMMARY

There is a strong correlation between glucose metabolism abnormalities and HF, with a bidirectional link between these 2 conditions, where glucose metabolism abnormalities at every step can affect HF. On the other hand, DM and IR are more prevalent in HF patients, and patients with both HF and DM have a worse prognosis, because of a combination of effects of both the components. Well known is the role of some new drugs in reducing the mortality in HF patients with DM, but more studies are warranted to know the real effect of treatment of IR in patients with HF.

REFERENCES

1. Ponikowski P, Voors AA, Anker SD, et al, ESC Scientific Document Group. 2016 ESC Guidelines for the diagnosis and treatment of acute and chronic heart failure: The Task Force for the Diagnosis and Treatment of Acute and Chronic Heart Failure of the European Society of Cardiology (ESC) developed with the special contribution of the Heart Failure Association (HFA) of the ESC. Eur Heart J 2016;37(27): 2129–200.

2. Mosterd A, Hoes AW. Clinical epidemiology of heart failure. Heart 2007;93(9):1137–46.

3. Redfield MM, Jacobsen SJ, Burnett JC Jr, et al. Burden of systolic and diastolic ventricular dysfunction in the community. JAMA 2003;289(2):194.

4. Bleumink GS, Knetsch AM, Sturkenboom MCJM, et al. Quantifying the heart failure epidemic: prevalence, incidence rate, lifetime risk and prognosis of heart failure - the Rotterdam Study. Eur Heart J 2004;25(18):1614–9.

5. Ceia F, Fonseca C, Mota T, et al. Prevalence of chronic heart failure in Southwestern Europe: the EPICA study. Eur J Heart Fail 2002;4(4):531–9.

6. Rydén L, Grant PJ, Anker SD, et al. ESC guidelines on diabetes, pre-diabetes, and cardiovascular diseases developed in collaboration with the EASD. Eur Heart J 2013;34(39):3035–87.

7. Bossone E, Arcopinto M, Iacoviello M, et al. Multiple hormonal and metabolic deficiency syndrome in chronic heart failure: rationale, design, and demographic characteristics of the T.O.S.CA. registry. Intern Emerg Med 2018;13(5):661–71.

8. Saccà L. Heart failure as a multiple hormonal deficiency syndrome. Circ Heart Fail 2009;2(2):151–6.

9. Arcopinto M, Salzano A, Isgaard J, et al. Hormone replacement therapy in heart failure. Curr Opin Cardiol 2015;30(3):277–84.

10. Cittadini A, Napoli R, Monti MG, et al. Metformin prevents the development of chronic heart failure in the SHHF rat model. Diabetes 2012;61(4):944–53.

11. Ingelsson E, Sundström J, Ärnlöv J, et al. Insulin resistance and risk of congestive heart failure. JAMA 2005;294(3):334.

12. Suskin N, McKelvie RS, Burns RJ, et al. Glucose and insulin abnormalities relate to functional capacity in patients with congestive heart failure. Eur Heart J 2000;21(16):1368–75.

13. Doehner W, Rauchhaus M, Ponikowski P, et al. Impaired insulin sensitivity as an independent risk factor for mortality in patients with stable chronic heart failure. J Am Coll Cardiol 2005;46(6):1019–26.

14. Wong AKF, Symon R, Alzadjali MA, et al. The effect of metformin on insulin resistance and exercise parameters in patients with heart failure. Eur J Heart Fail 2012;14(11):1303–10.

15. The Expert Committee on the Diagnosis and Classification of Diabetes Mellitus. Report of the expert committee on the diagnosis and classification of diabetes mellitus. Diabetes Care 1997;20:1183–97.

16. Genuth S, Alberti KGMM, Bennett P, et al, Expert Committee on the Diagnosis and Classification of Diabetes Mellitus. Follow-up report on the diagnosis of diabetes mellitus. Diabetes Care 2003;26(11):3160–7.

17. American Diabetes Association. Diagnosis and classification of diabetes mellitus. Diabetes Care 2012;35(suppl. 1). https://doi.org/10.2337/dc12-s064.

18. Tang Q, Li X, Song P, et al. Optimal cut-off values for the homeostasis model assessment of insulin resistance (HOMA-IR) and pre-diabetes screening: Developments in research and prospects for the future. Drug Discov Ther 2015;9(6):380–5.

19. Himsworth HP. Diabetes mellitus: its differentiation into insulin-sensitive and insulin-insensitive types. 1936. Int J Epidemiol 2013;42(6):1594–8.

20. Alebić MŠ, Bulum T, Stojanović N, et al. Definition of insulin resistance using the homeostasis model assessment (HOMA-IR) in IVF patients diagnosed with polycystic ovary syndrome (PCOS) according to the Rotterdam criteria. Endocrine 2014;47(2):625–30.

21. American Diabetes Association. Diagnosis and classification of diabetes mellitus. Diabetes Care 2010;33(suppl. 1). https://doi.org/10.2337/dc10-S062.

22. Marques-Vidal P, Mazoyer E, Bongard V, et al. Prevalence of insulin resistance syndrome in southwestern France and its relationship with inflammatory and hemostatic markers. Diabetes Care 2002;25(8):1371–7.

23. Radikova Z, Koska J, Huckova M, et al. Insulin sensitivity indices: a proposal of cut-off points for simple identification of insulin-resistant subjects. Exp Clin Endocrinol Diabetes 2006;114(5):249–56.

24. Geloneze B, Repetto EM, Geloneze SR, et al. The threshold value for insulin resistance (HOMA-IR) in an admixtured population. IR in the Brazilian Metabolic Syndrome Study. Diabetes Res Clin Pract 2006;72(2):219–20.

25. Esteghamati A, Ashraf H, Khalilzadeh O, et al. Optimal cut-off of homeostasis model assessment of insulin resistance (HOMA-IR) for the diagnosis of metabolic syndrome: third national surveillance of risk factors of non-communicable diseases in Iran (SuRFNCD-2007). Nutr Metab (Lond) 2010;7:26.

26. Yamada C, Moriyama K, Takahashi E. Optimal cut-off point for homeostasis model assessment of insulin resistance to discriminate metabolic syndrome in non-diabetic Japanese subjects. J Diabetes Investig 2012;3(4):384–7.

27. Yin J, Li M, Xu L, et al. Insulin resistance determined by homeostasis model assessment (HOMA) and associations with metabolic syndrome among Chinese children and teenagers. Diabetol Metab Syndr 2013;5(1):71.

28. Timoteo AT, Miranda F, Carmo MM, et al. Optimal cut-off value for homeostasis model assessment (HOMA) index of insulin-resistance in a population of patients admitted electively in a Portuguese cardiology ward. Acta Med Port 2014;27(4):473–9.

29. Hossain P, Kawar B, El Nahas M. Obesity and diabetes in the developing world — a growing challenge. N Engl J Med 2007;356(3):213–5.

30. Perrone-Filardi P, Paolillo S, Costanzo P, et al. The role of metabolic syndrome in heart failure. Eur Heart J 2015;36(39):2630–4.

31. Barzilay JI, Kronmal RA, Gottdiener JS, et al. The association of fasting glucose levels with congestive heart failure in diabetic adults ≥65 years: the cardiovascular health study. J Am Coll Cardiol 2004;43(12):2236–41.

32. Moller DE, Flier JS. Insulin resistance: mechanisms, syndromes, and implications. N Engl J Med 1991;325:938–48.

33. Pocock SJ, Wang D, Pfeffer MA, et al. Predictors of mortality and morbidity in patients with chronic heart failure. Eur Heart J 2006;27(1):65–75.

34. Paolillo S, Rengo G, Pellegrino T, et al. Insulin resistance is associated with impaired cardiac sympathetic innervation in patients with heart failure. Eur Heart J Cardiovasc Imaging 2015;16(10):1148–53.

35. Soläng L, Malmberg K, Rydén L. Diabetes mellitus and congestive heart failure. Further knowledge needed. Eur Heart J 1999;20(11):789–95.

36. Stratmann B, Tschoepe D. Heart in diabetes: not only a macrovascular disease. Diabetes Care 2011;34(suppl. 2). https://doi.org/10.2337/dc11-s208.

37. Stanley WC, Lopaschuk GD, Mccormack JG. Regulation of energy substrate metabolism in the diabetic heart. Cardiovasc Res 1997;34(1):25–33.

38. Dhalla NS, Liu X, Panagia V, et al. Subcellular remodeling and heart dysfunction in chronic diabetes. Cardiovasc Res 1998;40(2):239–47.

39. Rengo G, Pagano G, Paolillo S, et al. Impact of diabetes mellitus on lymphocyte GRK2 protein levels in patients with heart failure. Eur J Clin Invest 2015; 45(2):187–95.

40. Thrainsdottir I, Aspelund T, Thorgeirsson G, et al. The association between glucose abnormalities and heart failure in the population-based Reykjavik study. Diabetes Care 2005;28:612–6.

41. Bertoni AG, Hundley WG, Massing MW, et al. Heart failure prevalence, incidence, and mortality in the elderly with diabetes. Diabetes Care 2004;27(3): 699–703.

42. Kengne AP, Turnbull F, MacMahon S. The Framingham study, diabetes mellitus and cardiovascular disease: turning back the clock. Prog Cardiovasc Dis 2010;53(1):45–51.

43. He J, Ogden LG, Bazzano LA, et al. Risk factors for congestive heart failure in US men and women: NHANES I epidemiologic follow-up study. Arch Intern Med 2001;161(7):996–1002.

44. MacDonald MR, Petrie MC, Hawkins NM, et al. Diabetes, left ventricular systolic dysfunction, and chronic heart failure. Eur Heart J 2008;29(10): 1224–40.

45. Vaur L, Gueret P, Lievre M, et al. Development of congestive heart failure in type 2 diabetic patients with microalbuminuria or proteinuria: observations from the DIABHYCAR (type 2 DIABetes, Hypertension, CArdiovascular Events and Ramipril) study. Diabetes Care 2003;26(3):855–60. Available at: http://www.ncbi.nlm.nih.gov/pubmed/12610049.

46. Domanski M, Krause-Steinrauf H, Deedwania P, et al. The effect of diabetes on outcomes of patients with advanced heart failure in the BEST trial. J Am Coll Cardiol 2003;42(5):914–22.

47. Deedwania PC, Giles TD, Klibaner M, et al. Efficacy, safety and tolerability of metoprolol CR/XL in patients with diabetes and chronic heart failure: experiences from MERIT-HF. Am Heart J 2005;149(1): 159–67.

48. Gargiulo P, Savarese G, D'Amore C, et al. Efficacy and safety of glucagon-like peptide-1 agonists on macrovascular and microvascular events in type 2 diabetes mellitus: a meta-analysis. Nutr Metab Cardiovasc Dis 2017;27(12):1081–8.

49. Zinman B, Wanner C, Lachin JM, et al. Empagliflozin, cardiovascular outcomes, and mortality in type 2 diabetes. N Engl J Med 2015;373: 2117–28.

50. Butler J, Hamo CE, Filippatos G, et al. The potential role and rationale for treatment of heart failure with sodium – glucose co-transporter 2 inhibitors. Eur J Heart Fail 2017;19:1390–400.

Diabetic Cardiomyopathy
Definition, Diagnosis, and Therapeutic Implications

Stefania Paolillo, MD, PhD[a],*, Fabio Marsico, MD, PhD[b,c],
Maria Prastaro, MD[b], Francesco Renga, MD[b],
Luca Esposito, MD[b], Fabiana De Martino, MD[b],
Pierfrancesco Di Napoli, MD[b], Immacolata Esposito, MD[b],
Antonio Ambrosio, MD[b], Monica Ianniruberto, MS[b],
Rosa Mennella, MS[b], Roberta Paolillo[b],
Paola Gargiulo, MD, PhD[a]

KEYWORDS

- Diabetic cardiomyopathy • Diabetes mellitus • Heart failure • Systolic dysfunction
- Diastolic dysfunction

KEY POINTS

- Diabetic cardiomyopathy refers to a cardiac dysfunction observed in patients with diabetes that occurs in absence of other cardiovascular disease, such as coronary artery disease, hypertension, valvular, and congenital heart disease.
- The main metabolic abnormalities promoting cardiac dysfunction are the resistance to the metabolic actions of insulin in heart tissue, compensatory hyperinsulinemia, and the progression of hyperglycemia.
- Two stages of diabetic cardiomyopathy are described: an early stage characterized by left ventricular hypertrophy and impaired diastolic function, and a late stage characterized by cardiac fibrosis and systolic dysfunction.
- The occurrence of HF in patients affected by DM significantly impacts on quality of life, manifestation of new symptoms and worsening of existing symptoms, and on long-term prognosis.
- No target treatments have been tested in diabetic cardiomyopathy, thus clinical trials are needed to define the role of available HF therapies or to find new therapeutic targets for this clinical condition.

INTRODUCTION

A strict bidirectional relationship exists between diabetes mellitus (DM) and heart failure (HF). DM is common in HF patients with a prevalence range from 10% to 30%, and up to 40% in hospitalized HF subjects,[1] and adversely influences long-term morbidity and mortality of symptomatic and asymptomatic HF patients.[2] Conversely, HF is a common cardiovascular disease in patients affected by DM; the Framingham Heart Study showed that the occurrence of HF was twice as high in men with diabetes and five times higher in women with diabetes compared with control

Disclosure Statement: The authors have nothing to disclose.
Funding: Dr S. Paolillo is financed by the Italian Ministry of Health (Project Code: GR-2011–02354285).
[a] IRCCS SDN, Via Gianturco 113, Naples 80142, Italy; [b] Department of Advanced Biomedical Sciences, Section of Cardiology, Federico II University of Naples, Via Sergio Pansini, 5, Naples 80131, Italy; [c] Center for Congenital Heart Disease, University Hospital Inselspital, University of Bern, Freiburrgstrasse 18, Bern 3010, Switzerland
* Corresponding author. Via Gianturco, 113, Naples 80142, Italy.
E-mail address: stefania.paolillo@unina.it

Heart Failure Clin 15 (2019) 341–347
https://doi.org/10.1016/j.hfc.2019.02.003

subjects.[3] Analysis of data from 9.591 type 2 DM patients included in the Kaiser Permanente Northwest Division revealed HF in 11.8% of subjects with diabetes at baseline, with an additional 7.7% of patients developing HF during a 30-month period of observation.[4]

In particular, two distinct forms of HF might be observed in patients with diabetes. The first one is a typical systolic dysfunction consequent to coronary artery disease with no large differences with the general population; the other one is a typical manifestation of DM known as diabetic cardiomyopathy, a distinctive HF form observed in the diabetic population.

This review summarizes the characteristics of diabetic cardiomyopathy to better understand its pathophysiology and clinical manifestation and to analyze its prognostic relevance and therapeutic implication for a better management of subjects with diabetes.

DIABETIC CARDIOMYOPATHY: DEFINITION AND PATHOPHYSIOLOGY

The key problem is the absence of a universally accepted definition of diabetic cardiomyopathy, which makes studies of epidemiology, pathophysiology, and clinical characteristics and outcomes challenging. The first clinical description of diabetic cardiomyopathy appeared in literature in 1972 by Rubler and colleagues,[5] which reported postmortem data of four patients with diabetes who died of HF without evidence of hypertension, myocardial ischemia, or congenital or valvular heart disease. In the last position statement of the European Society of Cardiology on the management of DM and HF,[6] the authors report that the most commonly accepted definition of diabetic cardiomyopathy refers to a cardiac dysfunction observed in patients with diabetes that occurs in absence of all other cardiovascular disease, such as coronary artery disease, uncontrolled hypertension, significant valvular heart disease, and congenital heart disease.

The pathophysiology of diabetic cardiomyopathy is still under investigation; however, in the last years a wide variety of mechanisms have been suggested to be involved in this clinical condition, with most studies conducted in animals rather than humans. The main metabolic abnormalities promoting all the mechanisms leading to cardiac dysfunction are resistance to the metabolic actions of insulin in heart tissue (eg, insulin resistance), compensatory hyperinsulinemia, and progression of hyperglycemia. All these abnormalities lead to change in substrate metabolism and cardiac lipotoxicity, advanced glycated end-products (AGE) deposition, endothelial and microvascular dysfunction, inappropriate neurohormonal response, oxidative stress, and subcellular components abnormalities, as described in **Fig. 1**.

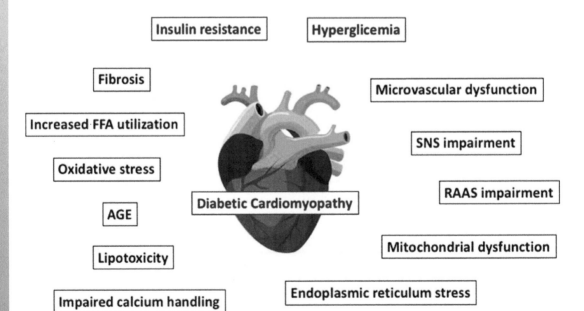

Fig. 1. Potential mechanisms implicated in the pathophysiology of diabetic cardiomyopathy. The main metabolic abnormalities promoting all the mechanisms leading to cardiac dysfunction are insulin resistance and hyperglycemia. See text for further details. FFA, free-fatty acid; RAAS, renin-angiotensin-aldosterone system; SNS, sympathetic nervous system.

Change in Substrate Metabolism and Cardiac Lipotoxicity

Under physiologic conditions, the heart can use fatty acids and glucose as energy substrates, a condition known as metabolic flexibility. In patients with DM, the reduced glucose uptake consequent to systemic and cardiac insulin resistance facilitates a substrate shift toward increased free fatty acid oxidation, resulting in reduced cardiac efficiency and in the loss of the metabolic flexibility of the heart.[7] Excessive accumulation of fatty acids in cardiac tissue and the associated lipotoxicity impairs insulin signaling leading to morphologic and structural abnormalities. All these conditions are responsible for an increase in myocardial oxygen consumption, an increase in the metabolic stress, and a significant reduction of cardiac efficiency and function.[8]

Advanced Glycated End-Products Deposition

AGE are proteins or lipids that become glycated after exposure to sugars, altering their functional features. AGE could exert a pivotal role in the development and progression of diabetic cardiomyopathy because they stimulate collagen expression and accumulation leading to the development of myocardial fibrosis with an increase in myocardial stiffness and a reduced cardiac compliance.[9]

Endothelial and Microvascular Dysfunction

Impaired endothelial function is a typical finding in diabetic cardiomyopathy. Patients with diabetes with and without coronary artery disease show significantly impaired peripheral vascular function compared with patients without diabetes without coronaropathy.[10] In particular, endothelial dysfunction in patients with diabetes without coronary artery disease is comparable with that of patients with coronary artery disease but without DM.[10] Moreover, in most patients with diabetes, microvascular dysfunction is associated with normal myocardial perfusion.[11] In the early stages of insulin resistance and diabetic cardiomyopathy, nitric oxide–induced vasodilatation is impaired, whereas endothelium-dependent vasodilatation is generally preserved. However, in the later stages, both mechanisms of vasodilatation may become impaired, promoting microvascular dysfunction and inflammation.[12]

Inappropriate Neurohormonal Response

Hyperinsulinemia, which characterizes the status of insulin resistance, promotes sympathetic activation.[13] Significantly more impaired cardiac sympathetic nervous system activity has been reported in HF patients with diabetes compared with HF subjects without diabetes[14] and associated with unfavorable clinical outcome.[15] Moreover, insulin resistance is associated with impaired cardiac adrenergic innervation also in absence of overt DM.[16] Activation of the adrenergic system increases β_1-adrenergic expression and signaling, promoting myocyte hypertrophy, interstitial fibrosis, myocyte apoptosis, and contractile dysfunction.[17] Similarly, increased activation of the renin-angiotensin-aldosterone system in states of insulin resistance or hyperinsulinemia promotes a remodeling processes in the heart.[17]

All the described mechanisms together with subcellular components abnormalities, because of mitochondrial dysfunction, endoplasmic reticulum stress, and impaired calcium handling, contribute to the occurrence and progression of diabetic cardiomyopathy and might represent in the next future potential new therapeutic targets.

DIABETIC CARDIOMYOPATHY: CLINICAL CHARACTERISTICS AND DIAGNOSIS

Diabetic cardiomyopathy was initially described as a dilated phenotype with eccentric left ventricular remodeling and systolic dysfunction.[5] However, in the last years a distinct phenotype from dilatative cardiomyopathy has been identified. Specifically, diabetic cardiomyopathy is defined as a condition characterized by a restrictive phenotype with left ventricular hypertrophy and diastolic dysfunction. Traditionally two stages of diabetic cardiomyopathy have been identified: an early stage characterized by left ventricular concentric hypertrophy, increased myocardial stiffness, increase in atrial filling pressure, and impaired diastolic function; and a late stage characterized by increase in cardiac fibrosis, further impairment in diastolic function, and appearance of systolic dysfunction (**Table 1**). However, a paper from Seferovic and Paulus[18] proposed that there are probably two distinct phenotypes of diabetic cardiomyopathy rather than successive stages of the same disease: a restrictive/HF with preserved ejection fraction (HFpEF) phenotype and a dilated/HF with reduced ejection fraction (HFrEF) phenotype. The distinction of these two forms might have important prognostic and therapeutic implications, because in the setting of HF there are several efficacious pharmacologic treatments for dilated/HFrEF, but still little evidence for the treatment of restrictive/HFpEF.[19]

The diagnosis of diabetic cardiomyopathy is still difficult because no clear definition for the disease is available, thus no clear diagnostic criteria have

Table 1
Pathophysiologic and clinical stages of diabetic cardiomyopathy

Stage	Pathophysiologic Findings	Clinical Findings
Early stage	Hyperglycemia and insulin resistance; increase in FFA, impaired calcium handling, impairment of SNS and RAAS, inflammatory response, AGE deposition	LV concentric hypertrophy Diastolic dysfunction Increase in left atrial filling pressure
Advanced stage	Cardiac fibrosis, cardiomyocyte apoptosis, microvascular and endothelial dysfunction, neurohormonal impairment, hyperactivation of the inflammatory response	Diastolic dysfunction Systolic dysfunction eventually LV dilation

Abbreviations: FFA, free-fatty acid; LV, left ventricle; RAAS, renin-angiotensin-aldosterone system; SNS, sympathetic nervous system.

been described. Patients usually complain of dyspnea and/or peripheral edema and the presence of signs of congestive HF need always to be investigated. Independently from the phenotype, the diagnosis requires the exclusion of coronary artery disease, significant valvular abnormalities, congenital heart disease, or hypertensive heart disease with the use of appropriate diagnostic techniques. Echocardiography is a fundamental tool for the initial assessment of a patient with suspected diabetic cardiomyopathy. In the early stage of the disease, or in the restrictive HFpEF form,[18] the typical echo findings are left ventricular normal diameters and volumes with concentric hypertrophy, preserved systolic function (with EF $\geq$50%), and evidence of diastolic dysfunction.

Use of cardiac MRI is under investigation in the setting of diabetic cardiomyopathy. In particular, the use of T1 mapping is an early approach to identify signs of diabetic cardiomyopathy because significant differences in myocardial extracellular matrix have been found comparing patients with diabetes with control subjects.[20]

The use of biomarkers in the diagnosis of diabetic cardiomyopathy is still not clear. Natriuretic peptides do not have a defined role in this context because of their poor positive predictive value for diastolic dysfunction and HFpEF.[18] Other biomarkers are currently under investigation. A study by Shaver and colleagues[21] demonstrated in 100 patients that a panel of biomarkers associated with echocardiography plays an important role in the detection of diabetic cardiomyopathy before the occurrence of clinical manifestation and irreversible complications. Specifically, the authors showed that early stages of diabetic cardiomyopathy are characterized by elevated levels of inflammatory markers; decreased levels antioxidant markers; and increased levels of markers of fibrosis, such as transforming growth factor-β.[21] Similarly, other markers of fibrosis, such as

procollagen type I propeptide and matrix metalloproteinase-7, are high in patients with diabetes with diastolic dysfunction.[22,23]

In the advanced stage of the disease, or in the dilated/HFrEF form,[18] these initial findings are typically accompanied by the occurrence of systolic dysfunction (ejection fraction <50%) together with an increase in left ventricular volumes.

DIABETIC CARDIOMYOPATHY: PROGNOSTIC AND THERAPEUTIC IMPLICATIONS

The strict bidirectional relationship between DM and HF exerts its effects also regarding prognostic implications. The occurrence of HF or diabetic cardiomyopathy in patients affected by DM significantly impacts quality of life, manifestation of new symptoms and worsening of existing symptoms, and long-term prognosis. The REACH Registry[24] analyzed the outcomes at 4 years of a cohort of 45.227 patients, of which 19.699 were affected by DM. The authors reported that DM was associated with a 33% greater risk of hospitalization for HF (9.4% vs 5.9%; adjusted odds ratio, 1.33; 95% confidence interval [CI], 1.18–1.50) and that in these patients the presence of HF at baseline was independently associated with cardiovascular death (adjusted HR, 2.45; 95% CI, 2.17–2.77; P<.001) and hospitalization for HF (adjusted odds ratio, 4.72; 95% CI, 4.22–5.29; P<.001).[24] Thus, patients with DM and HF are at particularly elevated risk of cardiovascular death.

However, the occurrence of DM in patients affected by HF might be responsible for disease progression and significantly impact long-term prognosis. A recent subanalysis of the PARADIGM-HF trial[25] conducted in 8.399 patients with HFrEF reported that patients with a history of DM (n = 2.907) had a higher risk of the primary composite outcome of HF hospitalization or cardiovascular mortality compared with those without

DM (adjusted hazard ratio, 1.38; 95% CI, 1.25–1.52; $P<.001$). Moreover, also patients with prediabetes (hemoglobin A_{1c} between 6.0% and 6.4%) were at higher risk (hazard ratio, 1.27; 95% CI, 1.10–1.47; $P<.001$) compared with those defined as at normal glycemic status (hemoglobin A_{1c} <6.0%).[25]

Regarding potential therapeutic approaches, no target treatments have been tested in the specific setting of diabetic cardiomyopathy, thus clinical trials are needed to define the role of available HF therapies or to find new therapeutic targets for this clinical condition.

Some preliminary studies of both treatment and prevention of myocardial abnormalities have been conducted in animals leading to interesting results. In an experimental model of diabetic cardiomyopathy, fenofibrate had a mild beneficial action on myocardial damage because it reduced fibrosis and fat (triacylglycerol) accumulation in the heart; metformin was more effective than fenofibrate in reducing fat content, however, with no effect on the reduction of fibrosis.[26] Similarly, trientine, a copper-selective chelator, improved cardiac function in rats with diabetes with significant left ventricular impairment.[27] As regards prevention of diabetic cardiomyopathy, experimental models of DM reported beneficial effects in protecting against myocardial damage for zinc supplementation,[28] AGE breakers (aminoguanidine),[29] angiotensin-converting enzyme inhibitors (captopril),[30] β-blockers (timolol),[31] and spironolactone.[32]

In humans, interesting data for the prevention of HF in patients with DM come from the results of clinical studies with Sodium-glucose cotransporter 2 (SGLT2) inhibitors. In particular, the EMPA-REG OUTCOME trial[33] demonstrated that treatment with empagliflozin reduced hospitalization for HF in patients with diabetes at high cardiovascular risk and that this effect was independent from the presence of HF at baseline.[34] The results of the study as regards HF outcomes were unexpected given that SGLT2 is not expressed in the heart and inhibition conferred beneficial cardiovascular effects that cannot be attributable to glucose-lowering alone. Even if the study population included patients with diabetes with different baseline cardiovascular profile, and the results cannot be generalized to diabetic cardiomyopathy, they widely stimulated the research to define the metabolic and molecular effects of empagliflozin in cardiovascular and renal protection.[35]

In animal studies, SGLT2 inhibitors slowed down atherosclerosis progression, and improved left ventricular negative remodeling and myocardial contractility.[36,37] Other potential mechanisms of cardiovascular protection with empagliflozin include the antioxidative, anti-inflammatory, and antiapoptotic effects observed in animal models, although evidence in humans is not yet available.[38] The mechanisms underlying cardiovascular protection with SGLT2 inhibitors are likely to be multifactorial, and outcome-specific trials (eg, involving patients with documented diabetic cardiomyopathy) will help gauge the value of new antidiabetics in the management of this specific clinical condition.

SUMMARY

Diabetic cardiomyopathy is a common and still underdiagnosed finding in patients with diabetes that may have a significant impact on quality of life, symptoms occurrence, and long-term prognosis.

The lack of a clear definition of this clinical condition makes the diagnosis difficult because no defined criteria are available. However, more attention should be focused on the research of cardiac abnormalities in patients with diabetes to avoid the progression to overt HF. Clinical trials are needed to clarify the therapeutic approach and to find new therapeutic targets for patients affected by diabetic cardiomyopathy.

ACKNOWLEDGMENTS

Dr. Roberta Paolillo is supported by a research grant from Cardiopath PhD program.

REFERENCES

1. Solang L, Malmberg K, Ryden L. Diabetes mellitus and congestive heart failure. Further knowledge needed. Eur Heart J 1999;20(11):789–95.
2. Shindler DM, Kostis JB, Yusuf S, et al. Diabetes mellitus, a predictor of morbidity and mortality in the Studies of Left Ventricular Dysfunction (SOLVD) Trials and Registry. Am J Cardiol 1996;77(11):1017–20.
3. Kannel WB, McGee DL. Diabetes and cardiovascular disease. The Framingham study. JAMA 1979;241(19):2035–8.
4. Nichols GA, Hillier TA, Erbey JR, et al. Congestive heart failure in type 2 diabetes: prevalence, incidence, and risk factors. Diabetes Care 2001;24(9):1614–9.
5. Rubler S, Dlugash J, Yuceoglu YZ, et al. New type of cardiomyopathy associated with diabetic glomerulosclerosis. Am J Cardiol 1972;30(6):595–602.
6. Seferovic PM, Petrie MC, Filippatos GS, et al. Type 2 diabetes mellitus and heart failure: a position statement from the Heart Failure Association of the

European Society of Cardiology. Eur J Heart Fail 2018;20(5):853–72.

7. Fang ZY, Prins JB, Marwick TH. Diabetic cardiomyopathy: evidence, mechanisms, and therapeutic implications. Endocr Rev 2004;25(4):543–67.

8. Jia G, DeMarco VG, Sowers JR. Insulin resistance and hyperinsulinaemia in diabetic cardiomyopathy. Nat Rev Endocrinol 2016;12(3):144–53.

9. Mandavia CH, Aroor AR, Demarco VG, et al. Molecular and metabolic mechanisms of cardiac dysfunction in diabetes. Life Sci 2013;92(11): 601–8.

10. Gargiulo P, Marciano C, Savarese G, et al. Endothelial dysfunction in type 2 diabetic patients with normal coronary arteries: a digital reactive hyperemia study. Int J Cardiol 2013;165(1):67–71.

11. Marciano C, Galderisi M, Gargiulo P, et al. Effects of type 2 diabetes mellitus on coronary microvascular function and myocardial perfusion in patients without obstructive coronary artery disease. Eur J Nucl Med Mol Imaging 2012;39(7):1199–206.

12. Vincent MA, Clerk LH, Lindner JR, et al. Microvascular recruitment is an early insulin effect that regulates skeletal muscle glucose uptake in vivo. Diabetes 2004;53(6):1418–23.

13. Anderson EA, Hoffman RP, Balon TW, et al. Hyperinsulinemia produces both sympathetic neural activation and vasodilation in normal humans. J Clin Invest 1991;87(6):2246–52.

14. Paolillo S, Rengo G, Pagano G, et al. Impact of diabetes on cardiac sympathetic innervation in patients with heart failure: a 123I meta-iodobenzylguanidine (123I MIBG) scintigraphic study. Diabetes Care 2013;36(8):2395–401.

15. Jacobson AF, Senior R, Cerqueira MD, et al. Myocardial iodine-123 meta-iodobenzylguanidine imaging and cardiac events in heart failure. Results of the prospective ADMIRE-HF (AdreView Myocardial Imaging for Risk Evaluation in Heart Failure) study. J Am Coll Cardiol 2010;55(20):2212–21.

16. Paolillo S, Rengo G, Pellegrino T, et al. Insulin resistance is associated with impaired cardiac sympathetic innervation in patients with heart failure. Eur Heart J Cardiovasc Imaging 2015;16(10): 1148–53.

17. Falcao-Pires I, Leite-Moreira AF. Diabetic cardiomyopathy: understanding the molecular and cellular basis to progress in diagnosis and treatment. Heart Fail Rev 2012;17(3):325–44.

18. Seferovic PM, Paulus WJ. Clinical diabetic cardiomyopathy: a two-faced disease with restrictive and dilated phenotypes. Eur Heart J 2015;36(27): 1718–27, 1727a-1727c.

19. Ponikowski P, Voors AA, Anker SD, et al. 2016 ESC Guidelines for the diagnosis and treatment of acute and chronic heart failure: the Task Force for the diagnosis and treatment of acute and chronic heart failure of the European Society of Cardiology (ESC). Developed with the special contribution of the Heart Failure Association (HFA) of the ESC. Eur J Heart Fail 2016;18(8):891–975.

20. Shang Y, Zhang X, Leng W, et al. Assessment of diabetic cardiomyopathy by cardiovascular magnetic resonance T1 mapping: correlation with left-ventricular diastolic dysfunction and diabetic duration. J Diabetes Res 2017;2017:9584278.

21. Shaver A, Nichols A, Thompson E, et al. Role of serum biomarkers in early detection of diabetic cardiomyopathy in the West Virginian population. Int J Med Sci 2016;13(3):161–8.

22. Ihm SH, Youn HJ, Shin DI, et al. Serum carboxy-terminal propeptide of type I procollagen (PIP) is a marker of diastolic dysfunction in patients with early type 2 diabetes mellitus. Int J Cardiol 2007;122(3): e36–8.

23. Ban CR, Twigg SM, Franjic B, et al. Serum MMP-7 is increased in diabetic renal disease and diabetic diastolic dysfunction. Diabetes Res Clin Pract 2010; 87(3):335–41.

24. Cavender MA, Steg PG, Smith SC Jr, et al. Impact of diabetes mellitus on hospitalization for heart failure, cardiovascular events, and death: outcomes at 4 years from the reduction of atherothrombosis for continued health (REACH) registry. Circulation 2015;132(10):923–31.

25. Kristensen SL, Preiss D, Jhund PS, et al. Risk related to pre-diabetes mellitus and diabetes mellitus in heart failure with reduced ejection fraction: insights from prospective comparison of ARNI With ACEI to determine impact on global mortality and morbidity in heart failure trial. Circ Heart Fail 2016;9(1) [pii: e002560].

26. Forcheron F, Basset A, Abdallah P, et al. Diabetic cardiomyopathy: effects of fenofibrate and metformin in an experimental model: the Zucker diabetic rat. Cardiovasc Diabetol 2009;8:16.

27. Lu J, Pontre B, Pickup S, et al. Treatment with a copper-selective chelator causes substantive improvement in cardiac function of diabetic rats with left-ventricular impairment. Cardiovasc Diabetol 2013;12:28.

28. Lu Y, Liu Y, Li H, et al. Effect and mechanisms of zinc supplementation in protecting against diabetic cardiomyopathy in a rat model of type 2 diabetes. Bosn J Basic Med Sci 2015;15(1):14–20.

29. Wu MS, Liang JT, Lin YD, et al. Aminoguanidine prevents the impairment of cardiac pumping mechanics in rats with streptozotocin and nicotinamide-induced type 2 diabetes. Br J Pharmacol 2008;154(4):758–64.

30. Rosen R, Rump AF, Rosen P. The ACE-inhibitor captopril improves myocardial perfusion in spontaneously diabetic (BB) rats. Diabetologia 1995; 38(5):509–17.

31. Turan B. A comparative summary on antioxidant-like actions of timolol with other antioxidants in diabetic cardiomyopathy. Curr Drug Deliv 2016;13(3):418–23.
32. Liu W, Gong W, He M, et al. Spironolactone protects against diabetic cardiomyopathy in streptozotocin-induced diabetic rats. J Diabetes Res 2018;2018:9232065.
33. Zinman B, Wanner C, Lachin JM, et al. Empagliflozin, cardiovascular outcomes, and mortality in type 2 diabetes. N Engl J Med 2015;373(22):2117–28.
34. Fitchett D, Zinman B, Wanner C, et al. Heart failure outcomes with empagliflozin in patients with type 2 diabetes at high cardiovascular risk: results of the EMPA-REG OUTCOME(R) trial. Eur Heart J 2016;37(19):1526–34.
35. Perrone-Filardi P, Avogaro A, Bonora E, et al. Mechanisms linking empagliflozin to cardiovascular and renal protection. Int J Cardiol 2017;241:450–6.
36. Tahara A, Kurosaki E, Yokono M, et al. Effects of SGLT2 selective inhibitor ipragliflozin on hyperglycemia, hyperlipidemia, hepatic steatosis, oxidative stress, inflammation, and obesity in type 2 diabetic mice. Eur J Pharmacol 2013;715(1–3):246–55.
37. Tate M, Grieve DJ, Ritchie RH. Are targeted therapies for diabetic cardiomyopathy on the horizon? Clin Sci (Lond) 2017;131(10):897–915.
38. Marx N, McGuire DK. Sodium-glucose cotransporter-2 inhibition for the reduction of cardiovascular events in high-risk patients with diabetes mellitus. Eur Heart J 2016;37(42):3192–200.

Metabolic Syndrome in Heart Failure: Friend or Foe?

Michele Arcopinto, MD[a], Alessandra Schiavo, MD[a], Andrea Salzano, MD[a,b], Eduardo Bossone, MD, PhD[c], Roberta D'Assante, PhD[d], Fabio Marsico, MD[e,f], Pablo Demelo-Rodriguez, MD, PhD[g,h], Ragavendra R. Baliga, MD, PhD[i], Antonio Cittadini, MD[a,j], Alberto M. Marra, MD[d,*]

KEYWORDS

- Metabolic syndrome • Heart failure • Insulin resistance • Risk stratification • Prognosis

KEY POINTS

- Metabolic syndrome is a cluster of cardiovascular risk factors that mirrors the presence of insulin resistance.
- Metabolic syndrome is associated with an increased risk of developing heart failure.
- Metabolic syndrome (and its components) seems to protect patients affected by heart failure with regards to mortality.

INTRODUCTION

Heart failure (HF) is a major health care issue insofar as it affects 3% of the general population and has become the main cause of mortality, hospitalization, and health care expenditures in individuals older than age 65 years.[1] According to population studies, the overall lifetime cost after HF diagnosis averages $109,541 per person, with more than 75% because of hospitalizations,[2] especially in the last months of life.[3] In the last two decades, growing attention was paid to find clusters of patients with an unfavorable disease progression deserving closer clinical attention and more aggressive treatment.

A consistent body of evidence demonstrated that patients with HF are burdened by several metabolic comorbidities that dramatically impact on outcomes.[4] Indeed, metabolic syndrome (MetS) is a cluster of cardiovascular (CV) risk factors mirroring the presence of insulin resistance (IR), such as central obesity, impaired glucose homeostasis, dyslipidemia, and systemic arterial hypertension. Epidemiologic data show that the relationship between MetS and HF is bidirectional. Patients with HF show a MetS phenotype in 22% to 68%[5–7]; however, the presence of MetS is associated with a two-fold likelihood risk of incident HF compared with the general population.[8,9]

Disclosure Statement: Dr A. Salzano receives research grant support from Cardiopath, UNINA, and Compagnia di San Paolo in the frame of Programme STAR. Dr A.M. Marra received institutional grant from Italian Healthcare Ministry (Ricerca Finalizzata per giovani ricercatori. Progetto n. GR-2016-02364727).

[a] Department of Translational Medical Sciences, "Federico II" University, Via Pansini 5, 80131 Naples, Italy; [b] Department of Cardiovascular Sciences, University of Leicester, Glenfield Hospital, Leicester, UK; [c] Cardiology Division, A Cardarelli Hospital, Via Antonio Cardarelli 9, 80131 Naples, Italy; [d] Istituto di Ricovero e Cura a Carattere Scientifico (IRCCS) SDN, Via Gianturco 113, 80142 Naples, Italy; [e] Department of Advanced Biomedical Sciences, Section of Cardiology, Federico II University of Naples, Via Pansini 5, 80131 Naples, Italy; [f] Center for Congenital Heart Disease, University Hospital "Inselspital," University of Bern, Bern, Switzerland; [g] Venous Thromboembolism Unit, Internal Medicine Department, Hospital General Universitario Gregorio Marañón, Calle del Dr. Esquerdo, 46, 28007 Madrid, Spain; [h] School of Medicine, Universidad Complutense de Madrid, Madrid, Spain; [i] Division of Cardiovascular Medicine, The Ohio State University Wexner Medical Center, Davis Heart and Lung Research Institute, 473 W 12th Avenue, Columbus, OH 43210, USA; [j] Interdisciplinary Research Centre in Biomedical Materials (CRIB), Via Pansini 5, 80131 Naples, Italy

* Corresponding author. Istituto di Ricovero e Cura a Carattere Scientifico (IRCCS) SDN, 113, Via Gianturco, 80143 Naples, Italy.
E-mail address: alberto_marra@hotmail.it

Heart Failure Clin 15 (2019) 349–358
https://doi.org/10.1016/j.hfc.2019.02.004

A complete understanding of the intricate interplay between MetS and HF is still an outstanding issue, the unravel of which may gather important information to clinicians with regards to prevention, prediction, and treatment optimization of HF. This review explores the existing association between MetS and HF by exploring the pathophysiologic link with IR, the current clinical implications in terms of prognostic association, and future research needs and opportunities.

METABOLIC SYNDROME: CLINICAL CONDITION OR RISK FACTORS COLLECTION?

Patients with MetS are characterized by a higher CV risk because of the contemporary presence of multiple risk factors in the same individual, such as obesity, arterial hypertension, dyslipidemias, and diabetes mellitus, any of which carries an increased CV risk.[10] In this view, it has been considered convenient to merge several risk factors under a unifying single entity so that a patient is easily labeled at higher CV risk. This is further reinforced by the concept that in all components of MetS, IR is a pivotal underlying mechanism. However, the definition of MetS relies on the presence or absence of certain criteria defined by prescriptive cutoffs: this facilitates the labeling of MetS, but it disperses more comprehensive information on the single risk factor and its contribution to the overall risk. Moreover, different definitions of MetS have been proposed by the main scientific communities, thus weakening comparisons about studies. Most common definitions are summarized in **Table 1**.

According to the different definitions, hallmarks of MetS are (1) abdominal obesity (measured by waist circumference or body mass index (BMI), (2) hypertriglyceridemia, (3) low high-density lipoprotein cholesterol, (4) arterial hypertension, and (5) impaired glucose metabolism. It is worth noting that noncardiac factors, such as liver disease (ie, nonalcoholic steatosis/hepatitis), renal disease, polycystic ovarian syndrome, and obstructive sleep apnea, may have independent or synergistic relationships with complementary cardiac MetS elements. Such factors, not accounted for in the current MetS definitions, are often related to others and may have an incremental adverse impact on CV outcome.[11]

METABOLIC SYNDROME AS A CLUSTER OF CLINICAL MANIFESTATIONS OF INSULIN RESISTANCE

Obesity in MetS is to be considered not as a mere fat accumulation, but as a dysfunction of the adipose tissue,[12,13] an endocrine organ able to synthetize several biologically active molecules and inflammatory mediators that ultimately lead to a state of loss in insulin-sensitivity.[14] IR results in decreased skeletal muscle glucose uptake and decreased inhibition of hepatic glucose output with increasing gluconeogenesis, which in turn contributes to hyperglycemia.[14] In turn, chronic hyperglycemia, often ending up in overt type 1 diabetes mellitus (T2DM), contributes to the process of nonenzymatic glycation and oxidation of proteins resulting in advanced glycation end-products (AGEs) formation. AGEs may further enhance IR by a variety of mechanisms, including synthesis of tumor necrosis factor-α, direct modification of the insulin molecule leading to an impairment of its action, and reduced peripheral insulin responsiveness.[15] The persistent hyperglycemia leads to sustained hyperinsulinemia resulting in a progressive reduction in pancreatic β-cell insulin secretion (β-cell exhaustion) in a population with genetical predisposition. This vicious cycle is considered the starting point for the clustering of all risk factors seen in MetS.[16]

The development of systemic arterial hypertension as a contributory factor in patients with MetS is less intuitively related to IR. However, hyperinsulinemia-induced sympathetic nervous system activation and other factors, such as endothelial dysfunction (caused by reactive oxygen species related, in turn, to increased generation of circulating free fatty acids), the inhibition of nitric oxide synthase, and the effects of adipose tissue–derived cytokines, all contribute to the development of arterial hypertension.[17] Moreover, because of overproduction of angiotensin II from hypertrophic adipocytes, the renin-angiotensin-aldosterone system is overactivated in obesity, which further increases arterial vasoconstriction. The consequent mineralocorticoid hormone overproduction is partially responsible for damage of the myocardial tissue seen in obese individuals.[18]

Taken together, the previously mentioned pathways lead to a chronic state of IR that finally culminates into the phenotypical manifestations of MetS.

METABOLIC SYNDROME AND RISK OF DEVELOPING HEART FAILURE

Several independent groups reported that MetS confers an increased risk of developing incident HF (**Table 2**). In 2006, the ULSAM longitudinal study was the first to report a three-fold increased risk to develop HF in a cohort of Swedish patients with MetS (first hospitalization for a cardiac

Table 1
Different definitions of metabolic syndrome

	WHO[66]	EGIR[67]	NCEPT/ATPIII[68]	IDF[69]
Year	1999	1999	2001	2005
Main criterion	IFG: fasting glucose level >110 mg/dL or IGT: glucose level >140 mg/dL 120 min after 75-g glucose oral load or T2DM plus ≥2 of the following	Hyperinsulinemia: fasting plasma insulin levels >75th percentile plus ≥3 of the following	≥3 of the following	Obesity (waist circumference) ≥94 cm for European men, ≥80 cm for European women, plus ≥2 of the following
Obesity	Waist/hip ratio >0.9 (men), >0.85 (women), and/or BMI >30 kg/m²	Waist circumference ≥94 cm (men), ≥80 cm (women)	Waist circumference ≥102 cm (men), ≥88 cm (women)	—
Dyslipidemia	HDL <35 mg/dL (men) (0.91 mmol/L) HDL <39 mg/dL (women) (<1.0 mmol/L) or Fasting TG ≥150 mg/dL (1.7 mmol/L)	HDL <39 mg/dL (1.0 mmol/L) or TG ≥177 mg/dL (2.0 mmol/L) or treatment	HDL <40 mg/dL (men) (1.0 mmol/L) HDL <50 mg/dL (women) (1.3 mmol/L) TG ≥150 mg/dL (1.69 mmol/L)	HDL <40 mg/dL (men) (<1.0 mmol/L) <50 mg/dL (women) (1.3 mmol/L) or treatment TG ≥150 mg/dL (1.7 mmol/L) or treatment
Hyperglycemia	—	FPG >6.1 mmol/L (110 mg/dL) Excluding T2DM	T2DM or IFG ≥110 mg/dL (6.1 mmol/L)	T2DM or IFG ≥100 mg/dL (5.6 mmol/L)
Hypertension	BP ≥140/90 mm Hg	BP ≥140/90 mm Hg or treatment	BP ≥130/85 mm Hg	SBP ≥130 mm Hg or DBP ≥85 mm Hg or treatment
Additional criteria	Microalbuminuria ≥20 μg/min or albumin/creatinine ≥30 mg/g	—	—	—

Abbreviations: BMI, body mass index; BP, blood pressure; DBP, diastolic blood pressure; EGIR, European Group for Study of Insulin Resistance; FPG, fasting plasma glucose; HDL, high-density lipoprotein cholesterol; IDF, International Diabetes Federation; IFG, impaired fasting glucose; IGT, impaired glucose tolerance; NCEPT/ATPIII, National Cholesterol Education Program-Adult Treatment Panel III; SBP, systolic blood pressure; T2DM, type 2 diabetes mellitus; TG, triglyceride; WHO, World Health Organization.

decompensation in patients with no history of cardiac disease).[19] The predictive value of MetS remained significant even when adjusted for already established HF risk factors (hypertension, diabetes, left ventricle [LV] hypertrophy, smoking habit, and BMI) (hazard ratio [HR], 1.66; P <0.05). The presence of an acute myocardial infarction during the follow-up further strengthened this relation (HR, 1.80; P<.05), thus providing insight into the pathophysiology of HF developing in MetS subjects.[19] These findings were substantially confirmed by the National Health and Nutrition Examination Survey III on 5549 North American men and nonpregnant women aged greater than 40 years.[8] According to this study, patients with MetS had an odds ratio of 1.8 of developing HF after adjustment for other risk factors (smoking habit, total cholesterol, LV hypertrophy, and electrocardiogram signs of possible myocardial infarction).[8]

Table 2
Risk of incident HF in patients with MetS

First Author, Year of Publication (Study Name)	Total Patients, n	Population and Follow-up	Study Design	Main Findings
Li et al,[8] 2007 (NHANES III)	5549	Men and nonpregnant women >40 y	Population-based, cross-sectional surveys	Participants with MetS were associated with about a 2-fold increased likelihood of self-reported CHF. In the multivariate model, the odds ratio of the MetS was no longer significant, suggesting that 90.7% of the association between the MetS and HF was attributed to the HOMA index (ie, insulin resistance).
Ingelsson et al,[19] 2006 (Uppsala Longitudinal Study of Adult Men)	2314	Men (age, >50 y) without HF, MI, or valvular disease at baseline were followed up for ≈20 y	Prospective study	The MetS increased the risk of developing HF >3-fold and remained significant after adjustment for established risk factors for HF in a multivariable Cox proportional hazards model.
Wang et al,[20] 2010	1032	Finns, aged 65–74 y at 20-y follow-up	Prospective study	Individual MetS components had HRs similar to that of the MetS as a whole in predicting incident HF, suggesting that the MetS does not predict HF better than its individual components. Moreover, the MetS predicts HF independently of MI, suggesting that it is also associated with nonischemic HF.
Bahrami et al,[10] 2008 (MESA study)	6814	People from US population (age 45–84 y)	Community-based multicenter cohort study	MetS predicts HF independently of MI, suggesting that it is also associated with nonischemic HF.

Abbreviations: CHF, congestive heart failure; HF, heart failure; HOMA, homeostasis model assessment; HR, hazard ratio; MESA study, Multi-Ethnic Study of Atherosclerosis; MetS, metabolic syndrome; MI, myocardial infarction; NHANES, National Health and Nutrition Examination Survey.

By adding the homeostasis model assessment index (a surrogate index for IR) to the model, the relationship between MetS and incident HF was markedly attenuated, leading to the observation that greater than 90% of the association was explained by the homeostasis model assessment index more than MetS per se.[8]

A 20-year follow-up study in elderly Finns confirmed that MetS increases the incidence of HF by a factor of 1.45 to 1.74 after adjustment for confounding risk factors. MetS was predictive of HF regardless of the cause (ischemic/nonischemic). However, the individual risk factors were predictive of HF as it was MetS itself, thus questioning its prognostic value over the traditional risk factors.[20] Other risk factors, related or not to the ones defining the MetS, may contribute to the overall HF risk in subjects with MetS. Among these, chronic inflammatory activity (elevated C-reactive protein) in the development of HF was able to increase the predictive value of MetS alone in the Cardiovascular Heart Study.[21]

In conclusion, available evidence is consistent to frame MetS as a powerful risk factor for incident HF. It seems less clear how stronger MetS is compared with individual CV risk factor and how MetS can improve the HF-prediction performance if supported by other emerging risk factors.

THE BIDIRECTIONAL INTERPLAY BETWEEN METABOLIC SYNDROME AND HEART FAILURE: IS INSULIN RESISTANCE THE PLAYER?

As demonstrated by a landmark prospective cohort study by Ingelsson and colleagues,[19] IR is a predictor of HF independently of diabetes and other established risk factors for HF. There are several possible explanations for the observed relationship. First, the aforementioned formation of AGEs, which leads to renin-angiotensin-aldosterone system activation, increased collagen cross-linking in the myocardium, and myocardial stiffness. Second, insulin may act as a growth factor in the myocardium. In fact, hyperinsulinemia leads to increased myocardial mass and decreased cardiac output as shown in animal studies.[22] Hyperinsulinemia leads to sodium retention,[23] which may lead to decompensation in subjects with otherwise subclinical myocardial dysfunction caused by volume expansion. Furthermore, hyperinsulinemia also leads to sympathetic nervous system activation,[24] which is a presumed causal factor for HF for its deleterious effects on cardiac structure and function, leading progressively to impaired cardiac innervations.[25–27] Finally, IR is related to an increased pressor response to angiotensin II[28]

and has recently been demonstrated to increase the stimulating effects of this hormone on cellular hypertrophy and collagen production,[29] leading to myocardial hypertrophy and fibrosis[30] and likely subsequent HF. However, HF is to be considered also an insulin-resistant metabolic state.[31] Arterial underfilling stimulates CV baroreceptors that activate sympathetic nervous system-mediated release of norepinephrine, to increase myocardial contractility and peripheral vascular resistance by activation of α - and β-adrenergic receptors.[32] Elevated plasma norepinephrine levels result in impaired insulin sensitivity and glucose tolerance.[33] Besides sympathetic overactivity, inflammatory activation, effects of HF drugs (β-blockers, angiotensin-converting enzyme inhibitors), and the reduced physical activity level might contribute to the development of IR in patients with HF without diabetes.[34,35] Animal studies show that glucose uptake is impaired by the occurrence of HF, probably caused by a reduced translocation of the glucose transporter GLUT4 on the cell membranes.[36] Because of the lack of intracellular glucose, cardiomyocytes begin to use free fatty acids, leading to a metabolic disadvantage. The resulting harmed energy production has detrimental consequences on the progression of the disease.[37] All these previously mentioned preclinical observations result in an increase risk to develop IR in patients with HF without diabetes.[38,39] Moreover, IR is clearly associated with survival in patients with HF.[40]

THE IMPACT OF METABOLIC SYNDROME ON HEART FAILURE OUTCOMES: A CASE OF "REVERSE EPIDEMIOLOGY"

The prognostic impact of MetS in HF is somewhat controversial. Most studies demonstrated that in patients with established diagnosis of HF, some established CV risk factors (hypertension, hypercholesterolemia, and obesity) display a protective effect on outcomes, a phenomenon also defined as "reverse epidemiology."[41–43] Such conditions are components of MetS. The impact of MetS (a clear risk factor for incident HF) has then been carefully explored in patients with established HF.

The impact MetS on HF outcomes was extensively studied by Perrone-Filardi and colleagues.[7] In this study patients with HF with MetS had a significantly reduced risk of all-cause death and death for HF compared with patients without MetS. The highest mortality rate was observed among patients with T2DM without MetS, whereas patients with MetS and T2DM had a similar mortality risk of patients without both conditions. These results are in line with those of Hassan and colleagues,[44] which reported a reduced mortality rate in patients with HF with MetS (adjusted HR, 0.73). However, a prospective study performed by Tamariz and coworkers[5] reported a 1.5-fold increase in mortality in patients with HF with MetS. **Table 3** summarizes studies aimed at evaluating the associations between MetS and mortality in patients with HF.

Landmark studies on chronic HF have demonstrated that BMI is inversely associated with long-term mortality: patients with higher BMI displayed lower mortality rates as compared with those with lower BMI, regardless of LV ejection fraction.[41,45] This so-called "obesity paradox" has not been fully elucidated. A potential explanation of this phenomenon is that a higher BMI may provide a greater protection against malnutrition-inflammation characterizing chronic HF and against cachexia related to end-stage HF.[46] Indeed, the presence of an anabolic overdrive in patients with HF seems to be protective against poor outcomes.[47–53] The obesity paradox has been also described in acute settings by Fonarow and colleagues,[46] in 108,927 patients hospitalized for acute HF.

An epidemiologic paradox also exists in the HF-hypertension relationship. Once advanced HF is manifest, a higher blood pressure is associated with a better prognosis as described in subanalysis from the Digitalis Investigation Group trial database[54] and from a meta-analysis of 10 studies.[55] In these studies, the average decrease in mortality rates associated with a 10 mm Hg higher systolic blood pressure was 13.0% in the HF population. As expected, HF-hypertension relationship is different in patients with mild versus severe HF, with a U-shaped relationship in the former group and a linear relationship in the latter.

There is no doubt that the presence of T2DM in patients with HF is associated with increased morbidity and mortality (1.3–2.0 additive risk), especially in those with ischemic cause.[56] Less

Table 3
Impact of MetS on survival in patients with established HF

First Author, Year of Publication	Total Patients, n	Setting	Main Findings
Hassan et al,[44] 2008	625	A retrospective cohort of patients admitted for HF	Lower mortality in patients with HF with MetS compared with those without MetS (43.8% vs 57.6%). There was a nonlinear decrease in mortality with an increasing number of MetS criteria: 68.2% in those with no criteria to 37.0% in those with all 5 criteria.
Tamariz et al,[5] 2009	865	A prospective cohort of outpatients with HFrEF (EF <40%)	Mortality of 24% in those with MetS compared with 16% in those without at 2.6 y of follow-up. The Kaplan-Meier curves were similar for up to 4 y of follow-up for both groups and diverged thereafter with higher mortality in the MetS group.
Perrone-Filardi et al,[7] 2015	6648	HF with MetS vs HF without MetS HF without MetS and without T2DM vs HF with MetS without T2DM	Risk of all-cause death and HF death was significantly reduced in patients with MetS. Risk of all-cause and HF death was significantly lower in patients with MetS and no T2DM.
		HF without MetS and without T2DM vs HF without MetS but with T2DM	Risk of all-cause and HF death was significantly increased in patients with T2DM and no MetS.

Abbreviations: EF, ejection fraction; GISSI-HF, Gruppo Italiano per lo Studio della Sopravvivenza nell'Insufficienza Cardiaca - heart failure; HF, heart failure; HFrEF, heart failure with reduced ejection fraction; MESA study, Multi-Ethnic Study of Atherosclerosis; MetS, metabolic syndrome; NHANES, National Health and Nutrition Examination Survey; T2DM, diabetes mellitus.

clear is how glycemic control (hemoglobin [Hb]A_{1c} target) impacts on HF outcomes. Some observational data have demonstrated a U-shaped or inverse relationship between HbA_{1c} and mortality in individuals with established HF and T2DM,[57] with most studies demonstrating that poorer prognosis was observed in patients with HF with strict glycemic control (HbA_{1c} <7%) compared with those with a more modest control (HbA_{1c} >7%). However, the absence of data from clinical trials of targeted glucose control in HF population entails insufficient evidence to recommend specific glucose treatment targets in such patients. As summarized in the next section, the scenario for diabetes control in patients with HF is currently changing and is expected to profoundly change for the recent introduction of novel molecules for T2DM treatment.

In patients with established HF, several analyses have demonstrated an inverse relationship between cholesterol levels and outcome: low cholesterol levels have been shown to be independently associated with increased mortality and higher cholesterol levels with improved survival.[58] Available evidence does not support the routine use of statins to treat HF and that it is not indicated outside the current practice guidelines for the primary and secondary prevention of atherosclerotic vascular disease.

TREATING METABOLIC ABNORMALITIES IN HEART FAILURE

Although there is no doubt about the importance of the control of metabolic risk factors to reduce the incidence of HF, more challenging is the management of MetS in patients with HF, because of the better outcome demonstrated in patients with HF and MetS compared with those without MetS in most studies. To date, guidelines suggest to implement weight loss only in more advanced obese patients (BMI, 35–45 kg/m^2).[59]

With regards to lipid abnormalities, n-3 polyunsaturated fatty acids are likely to improve morbidity and mortality in a large population of patients with symptomatic HF of any cause,[60] whereas statins did not improve the prognosis in patients with HF.[61,62]

The optimal antihyperglycemic therapy in patients with HF with T2DM has not been well defined. The wide therapeutic armamentarium for the treatment of T2DM includes insulin-sensitizers, insulin secretagogues, thiazolidinediones, recombinant insulins with a wide array of kinetics, incretins (glucagon-like peptide-1 agonists and dipeptidyl peptidase-4 inhibitors), and glycosurics (sodium-glucose cotransporter 2 inhibitors, gliflozins).

Because MetS is sustained by IR, insulin-sensitizers should supposedly have a prominent role for the treatment of this condition. Metformin was previously contraindicated in individuals with HF because of potential concerns about lactic acidosis. However, this adverse event is considered extremely rare and multiple observational studies in patients with established HF have suggested that metformin not only is safe but also may be associated with improved survival in patients with T2DM and HF with preserved renal function.[63] Second-generation sulfonylureas have shown neutral effects on HF outcomes but they are often not preferred in patients with HF for the risk of hypoglycemia and weight gain.[64] Many patients with diabetes mellitus and HF require insulin therapy either as monotherapy or in combination with other agents to achieve adequate glycemic control. Observational studies have demonstrated an association between insulin use and increased mortality, although these findings are potentially limited by the fact that patients on insulin therapy are more likely to have a longer T2DM duration and severity, with a higher CV risk.[31]

Although the incretin-based therapies could have potential benefit in HF, they have not been studied extensively in patients with established HF. Gliflozins represent the most novel drug class for diabetes therapy. Exciting data in registration trials (significant reduction in CV death, all-cause mortality, and HF hospitalizations)[65] paved the way for two large ongoing randomized controlled trial started in 2017 to test empaglifozin as a potential therapy on top of guideline-based therapy in HF, in patients with and without T2DM (NCT03057977, NCT03036124).

SUMMARY

The relationship between MetS and HF is still unclear and challenging. MetS confers an increase risk to develop incident HF and this effect seems to be mediated mainly by IR. However, MetS seems to be somehow protective in patients with already established HF, albeit IR might impair survival of patients with HF, whereas obesity without IR seems to be protective. IR and HF often coexist and more importance should be given to screening, prevention, and treatments of IR and diabetes mellitus, because they have been demonstrated to be the most important prognostic predictor of adverse outcome in patients with HF.

REFERENCES

1. Braunwald E. Heart failure. JACC Heart Fail 2013;1: 1–20.

2. Dunlay SM, Shah ND, Shi Q, et al. Lifetime costs of medical care after heart failure diagnosis. Circ Cardiovasc Qual Outcomes 2011;4:68–75.

3. Obi EN, Swindle JP, Turner SJ, et al. Health care costs for patients with heart failure escalate nearly 3-fold in final months of life. J Manag Care Spec Pharm 2016;22:1446–56.

4. Saccà L. Heart failure as a multiple hormonal deficiency syndrome. Circ Heart Fail 2009;2:151–6.

5. Tamariz L, Hassan B, Palacio A, et al. Metabolic syndrome increases mortality in heart failure. Clin Cardiol 2009;32:327–31.

6. Miura Y, Fukumoto Y, Shiba N, et al. Prevalence and clinical implication of metabolic syndrome in chronic heart failure. Circ J 2010;74:2612–21.

7. Perrone-Filardi P, Savarese G, Scarano M, et al. Prognostic impact of metabolic syndrome in patients with chronic heart failure: data from GISSI-HF trial. Int J Cardiol 2015;178:85–90.

8. Li C, Ford ES, McGuire LC, et al. Association of metabolic syndrome and insulin resistance with congestive heart failure: findings from the Third National Health and Nutrition Examination Survey. J Epidemiol Community Health 2007;61:67–73.

9. Ingelsson E, Sundström J, Arnlöv J, et al. Insulin resistance and risk of congestive heart failure. JAMA 2005;294:334–41.

10. Bahrami H, Bluemke DA, Kronmal R, et al. Novel metabolic risk factors for incident heart failure and their relationship with obesity: the MESA (Multi-Ethnic Study of Atherosclerosis) study. J Am Coll Cardiol 2008;51:1775–83.

11. Said S, Mukherjee D, Whayne TF. Interrelationships with metabolic syndrome, obesity and cardiovascular risk. Curr Vasc Pharmacol 2016;14:415–25.

12. Van Lookeren Campagne M, Oestreicher AB, Buma P, et al. Ultrastructural localization of adrenocorticotrophic hormone and the phosphoprotein B-50/growth-associated protein 43 in freeze-substituted, Lowicryl HM20-embedded mesencephalic central gray substance of the rat. Neuroscience 1991;42:517–29.

13. Oda E. The metabolic syndrome as a concept of adipose tissue disease. Hypertens Res 2008;31:1283–91.

14. Kostis JB, Sanders M. The association of heart failure with insulin resistance and the development of type 2 diabetes. Am J Hypertens 2005;18:731–7.

15. Song F, Schmidt AM. Glycation and insulin resistance: novel mechanisms and unique targets? Arterioscler Thromb Vasc Biol 2012;32:1760–5.

16. Kolovou GD, Anagnostopoulou KK, Cokkinos DV. Pathophysiology of dyslipidaemia in the metabolic syndrome. Postgrad Med J 2005;81:358–66.

17. Samson SL, Garber AJ. Metabolic syndrome. Endocrinol Metab Clin North Am 2014;43:1–23.

18. Putnam K, Shoemaker R, Yiannikouris F, et al. The renin-angiotensin system: a target of and contributor to dyslipidemias, altered glucose homeostasis, and hypertension of the metabolic syndrome. Am J Physiol Heart Circ Physiol 2012;302:H1219–30.

19. Ingelsson E, Arnlöv J, Lind L, et al. Metabolic syndrome and risk for heart failure in middle-aged men. Heart 2006;92:1409–13.

20. Wang J, Sarnola K, Ruotsalainen S, et al. The metabolic syndrome predicts incident congestive heart failure: a 20-year follow-up study of elderly Finns. Atherosclerosis 2010;210:237–42.

21. Suzuki T, Katz R, Jenny NS, et al. Metabolic syndrome, inflammation, and incident heart failure in the elderly: the cardiovascular health study. Circ Heart Fail 2008;1:242–8.

22. Holmäng A, Yoshida N, Jennische E, et al. The effects of hyperinsulinaemia on myocardial mass, blood pressure regulation and central haemodynamics in rats. Eur J Clin Invest 1996;26:973–8.

23. DeFronzo RA, Cooke CR, Andres R, et al. The effect of insulin on renal handling of sodium, potassium, calcium, and phosphate in man. J Clin Invest 1975;55:845–55.

24. Anderson EA, Hoffman RP, Balon TW, et al. Hyperinsulinemia produces both sympathetic neural activation and vasodilation in normal humans. J Clin Invest 1991;87:2246–52.

25. Rengo G, Perrone-Filardi P, Femminella GD, et al. Targeting the β-adrenergic receptor system through G-protein-coupled receptor kinase 2: a new paradigm for therapy and prognostic evaluation in heart failure: from bench to bedside. Circ Heart Fail 2012;5:385–91.

26. Paolillo S, Rengo G, Pellegrino T, et al. Insulin resistance is associated with impaired cardiac sympathetic innervation in patients with heart failure. Eur Heart J Cardiovasc Imaging 2015;16:1148–53.

27. Paolillo S, Rengo G, Pagano G, et al. Impact of diabetes on cardiac sympathetic innervation in patients with heart failure: a 123I meta-iodobenzylguanidine (123I MIBG) scintigraphic study. Diabetes Care 2013;36:2395–401.

28. Gaboury CL, Simonson DC, Seely EW, et al. Relation of pressor responsiveness to angiotensin II and insulin resistance in hypertension. J Clin Invest 1994;94:2295–300.

29. Sartori M, Ceolotto G, Papparella I, et al. Effects of angiotensin II and insulin on ERK1/2 activation in fibroblasts from hypertensive patients. Am J Hypertens 2004;17:604–10.

30. Bell DSH. Heart failure: the frequent, forgotten, and often fatal complication of diabetes. Diabetes Care 2003;26:2433–41.

31. Pocock SJ, Wang D, Pfeffer MA, et al. Predictors of mortality and morbidity in patients with chronic heart failure. Eur Heart J 2006;27:65–75.

32. Paolisso G, Riu S De, Marrazzo G, et al. Insulin resistance and hyperinsulinemia in patients with chronic congestive heart failure. Metabolism 1991;40:972–7.

33. Levine TB, Francis GS, Goldsmith SR, et al. Activity of the sympathetic nervous system and renin-angiotensin system assessed by plasma hormone levels and their relation to hemodynamic abnormalities in congestive heart failure. Am J Cardiol 1982; 49:1659–66.

34. Tenenbaum A, Fisman EZ. Impaired glucose metabolism in patients with heart failure: pathophysiology and possible treatment strategies. Am J Cardiovasc Drugs 2004;4:269–80.

35. Doehner W, Frenneaux M, Anker SD. Metabolic impairment in heart failure: the myocardial and systemic perspective. J Am Coll Cardiol 2014;64: 1388–400.

36. Nikolaidis LA, Sturzu A, Stolarski C, et al. The development of myocardial insulin resistance in conscious dogs with advanced dilated cardiomyopathy. Cardiovasc Res 2004;61:297–306.

37. Dutka DP, Pitt M, Pagano D, et al. Myocardial glucose transport and utilization in patients with type 2 diabetes mellitus, left ventricular dysfunction, and coronary artery disease. J Am Coll Cardiol 2006;48:2225–31.

38. Swan JW, Anker SD, Walton C, et al. Insulin resistance in chronic heart failure: relation to severity and etiology of heart failure. J Am Coll Cardiol 1997;30:527–32.

39. Suskin N, McKelvie RS, Burns RJ, et al. Glucose and insulin abnormalities relate to functional capacity in patients with congestive heart failure. Eur Heart J 2000;21:1368–75.

40. Doehner W, Rauchhaus M, Ponikowski P, et al. Impaired insulin sensitivity as an independent risk factor for mortality in patients with stable chronic heart failure. J Am Coll Cardiol 2005;46:1019–26.

41. Horwich TB, Fonarow GC. Glucose, obesity, metabolic syndrome, and diabetes. J Am Coll Cardiol 2010;55:283–93.

42. Kalantar-Zadeh K, Block G, Horwich T, et al. Reverse epidemiology of conventional cardiovascular risk factors in patients with chronic heart failure. J Am Coll Cardiol 2004;43:1439–44.

43. Yancy CW, Jessup M, Bozkurt B, et al. 2016 ACC/AHA/HFSA focused update on new pharmacological therapy for heart failure: an update of the 2013 ACCF/AHA guideline for the management of heart failure: a report of the American College of Cardiology/American Heart Association Task Force on clinical practice guidelines and the Heart Failure Society of America. Circulation 2016;134:e282–93.

44. Hassan SA, Deswal A, Bozkurt B, et al. The metabolic syndrome and mortality in an ethnically diverse heart failure population. J Card Fail 2008;14:590–5.

45. Davos CH, Doehner W, Rauchhaus M, et al. Body mass and survival in patients with chronic heart failure without cachexia: the importance of obesity. J Card Fail 2003;9:29–35.

46. Fonarow GC, Srikanthan P, Costanzo MR, et al, ADHERE Scientific Advisory Committee and Investigators. An obesity paradox in acute heart failure: analysis of body mass index and inhospital mortality for 108,927 patients in the Acute Decompensated Heart Failure National Registry. Am Heart J 2007; 153:74–81.

47. Arcopinto M, Isgaard J, Marra AM, et al. IGF-1 predicts survival in chronic heart failure. Insights from the T.O.S.CA. (Trattamento Ormonale Nello Scompenso CArdiaco) registry. Int J Cardiol 2014;176: 1006–8.

48. Arcopinto M, Salzano A, Giallauria F, et al, T.O.S.CA. (Trattamento Ormonale Scompenso CArdiaco) Investigators. Growth hormone deficiency is associated with worse cardiac function, physical performance, and outcome in chronic heart failure: insights from the T.O.S.CA. GHD study. PLoS One 2017;12:e0170058.

49. Jankowska EA, Biel B, Majda J, et al. Anabolic deficiency in men with chronic heart failure: prevalence and detrimental impact on survival. Circulation 2006; 114:1829–37.

50. Cittadini A, Bossone E, Marra AM, et al. Anabolic/catabolic imbalance in chronic heart failure. Monaldi Arch Chest Dis 2010;74:53–6 [in Italian].

51. Bossone E, Limongelli G, Malizia G, et al. The T.O.S.CA. Project: research, education and care. Monaldi Arch Chest Dis 2011;76(4):198–203.

52. Marra AM, Bobbio E, D'Assante R, et al. Growth hormone as biomarker in heart failure. Heart Fail Clin 2018;14:65–74.

53. Salzano A, Marra AM, Ferrara F, et al. Multiple hormone deficiency syndrome in heart failure with preserved ejection fraction. Int J Cardiol 2016; 225:1–3.

54. Lee TT, Chen J, Cohen DJ, et al. The association between blood pressure and mortality in patients with heart failure. Am Heart J 2006;151:76–83.

55. Raphael CE, Whinnett ZI, Davies JE, et al. Quantifying the paradoxical effect of higher systolic blood pressure on mortality in chronic heart failure. Heart 2008;95:56–62.

56. Targher G, Dauriz M, Laroche C, et al, ESC-HFA HF Long-Term Registry investigators. In-hospital and 1-year mortality associated with diabetes in patients with acute heart failure: results from the ESC-HFA Heart Failure Long-Term Registry. Eur J Heart Fail 2017;19:54–65.

57. Aguilar D, Bozkurt B, Ramasubbu K, et al. Relationship of hemoglobin A1C and mortality in heart failure patients with diabetes. J Am Coll Cardiol 2009;54: 422–8.

58. Pekkanen J, Linn S, Heiss G, et al. Ten-year mortality from cardiovascular disease in relation to cholesterol level among men with and without preexisting cardiovascular disease. N Engl J Med 1990;322: 1700–7.

59. Ponikowski P, Voors AA, Anker SD, et al. 2016 ESC Guidelines for the diagnosis and treatment of acute and chronic heart failure. Eur Heart J 2016;37: 2129–200.

60. Tavazzi L, Maggioni AP, Marchioli R, et al, Gissi-HF Investigators. Effect of n-3 polyunsaturated fatty acids in patients with chronic heart failure (the GISSI-HF trial): a randomised, double-blind, placebo-controlled trial. Lancet 2008;372:1223–30.

61. Kjekshus J, Apetrei E, Barrios V, et al, CORONA Group. Rosuvastatin in older patients with systolic heart failure. N Engl J Med 2007;357:2248–61.

62. GISSI-HF Investigators. Effect of rosuvastatin in patients with chronic heart failure (the GISSI-HF trial): a randomised, double-blind, placebo-controlled trial. Lancet 2008;372:1231–9.

63. Aguilar D, Chan W, Bozkurt B, et al. Metformin use and mortality in ambulatory patients with diabetes and heart failure. Circ Heart Fail 2011;4:53–8.

64. Masoudi FA. Thiazolidinediones, metformin, and outcomes in older patients with diabetes and heart failure: an observational study. Circulation 2005;111: 583–90.

65. Fitchett D, Zinman B, Wanner C, et al, EMPA-REG OUTCOME® Trial Investigators. Heart failure outcomes with empagliflozin in patients with type 2 diabetes at high cardiovascular risk: results of the EMPA-REG OUTCOME trial. Eur Heart J 2016;37: 1526–34.

66. Alberti KG, Zimmet PZ. Definition, diagnosis and classification of diabetes mellitus and its complications. Part 1: diagnosis and classification of diabetes mellitus provisional report of a WHO consultation. Diabet Med 1998;15:539–53.

67. Balkau B, Charles MA. Comment on the provisional report from the WHO consultation. European Group for the Study of Insulin Resistance (EGIR). Diabet Med 1999;16:442–3.

68. Expert Panel on Detection, Evaluation, and Treatment of High Blood Cholesterol in Adults. Executive summary of the third report of the National Cholesterol Education Program (NCEP) expert panel on detection, evaluation, and treatment of high blood cholesterol in adults (adult treatment panel III). JAMA 2001;285:2486–97.

69. Zimmet P, M M Alberti KG, Serrano Ríos M. A new international diabetes federation worldwide definition of the metabolic syndrome: the rationale and the results. Rev Esp Cardiol 2005;58:1371–6 [in Spanish].

Anemia and Iron Deficiency in Heart Failure
Clinical and Prognostic Role

Damiano Magrì, MD, PhD[a], Fabiana De Martino, MD[b],
Federica Moscucci, MD[c],
Piergiuseppe Agostoni, MD, PhD[b,d],*,
Susanna Sciomer, MD[c]

KEYWORDS

- Anemia • Hemoglobin • Iron deficiency • Cardiopulmonary exercise test • Heart failure

KEY POINTS

- Anemia is a highly prevalent comorbidity in heart failure (HF) patients and represents both a marker of HF severity and a predictor of poor prognosis.
- Anemia is per se associated with impaired exercise performance and functional capacity.
- Iron deficiency (ID) is an important comorbidity of HF, but the diagnosis and correction of ID remain largely unrecognized in the cardiology community.
- The presence of ID, irrespective of Hb levels, has been associated with a reduced peak oxygen uptake and an increased ventilation versus carbon dioxide production slope in patients with HF.
- Large randomized trials strongly support intravenous (IV) iron administration, a beneficial therapeutic strategy to be adopted in HF patients with ID, and guidelines also recommend IV iron replacement therapy in the HF patients who meet the ID criteria.

ANEMIA
Criteria, Prevalence, and Underlying Mechanisms in Heart Failure

Anemia represents a continuum; nonetheless it is arbitrarily defined by the World Health Organization (WHO) as hemoglobin (Hb) concentration less than 13 g/dL in men and less than 12 g/dL in women.

Anemia is a highly prevalent comorbidity in heart failure (HF) patients, ranging from 30% to 70% as reported in several studies[1–12] (**Table 1**). Although anemia is usually considered a possible HF consequence, it should be noted that, once established, it might act also as a significant determinant of its progression.[13] In patients with HF, anemia has a multifactorial cause (**Table 2**): it may be due to reduced intestinal iron absorption, caused by the reduced expression of hepcidin[14] and ferroportin in gut cells; as in every chronic condition, in HF patients there is an increased cytokine production (tumor necrosis factor alpha, in particular), which

Disclosure: The authors have nothing to disclose.
[a] Department of Clinical and Molecular Medicine, Azienda Ospedaliera Sant'Andrea, "Sapienza" Università degli Studi di Roma, Roma, Italy; [b] Department of "Scompenso Cardiaco e Cardiologia Clinica", Centro Cardiologico Monzino, IRCCS, Milano, Italy; [c] Dipartimento di Scienze Cardiovascolari, Respiratorie, Nefrologiche, Anestesiologiche e Geriatriche, "Sapienza" Università degli Studi di Roma, Roma, Italy; [d] Cardiovascular Section, Department of Clinical Sciences and Community Health, University of Milano, Centro Cardiologico Monzino, IRCCS, Via Parea 4, 20138 Milan, Italy
* Corresponding author. Cardiovascular Section, Department of Clinical Sciences and Community Health, Centro Cardiologico Monzino, IRCCS, Via Parea 4, 20138 Milan, Italy.
E-mail addresses: piergiuseppe.agostoni@ccfm.it; piergiuseppe.agostoni@unimi.it

Heart Failure Clin 15 (2019) 359–369
https://doi.org/10.1016/j.hfc.2019.02.005
1551-7136/19/© 2019 Elsevier Inc. All rights reserved.

Table 1
Major studies on heart failure, anemia, and prognosis

	Study Cohort	Variables	Mortality	Prognosis	Impact of Possible Treatments
Diez-Lopez et al,[4] 2016	1173 consecutive outpatients with HF	Hb g/dL (anemia as per WHO criteria)	Increased mortality	Worse prognosis	Iron/EPO supplementation did not improve outcomes Blood transfusions were related to poor prognosis
Van der Meer et al,[11] 2013	1969 pts with AHF and impaired renal function	Hb g/dL	Hb-concentration changes with better renal function predicted better 180-d survival	Worse prognosis in anemic patients with impaired renal function	Rapid response to diuretic therapy (hemoconcentration) in the first 4 d correlated with a better prognosis
Dvornik et al,[5] 2018	165 pts admitted for AHF	RDW (cutoff 16.4%)	Lower RDW correlated with better survival	Worse prognosis (predictor of in-hospital fatal outcome)	
Tseliou et al,[9] 2014	80 pts with stage D HF, recently decompensated	RDW	Anemia alone was associated with higher mortality	Worse prognosis. Lower RDW correlated with adverse outcome in pts with advanced-stage HF, recently decompensated	
Migone de Amicis,[8] 2017	719 pts (55.6%women) admitted for a first HF episode at hospital	Hb g/dL	Increased midterm (1 y) mortality. In-hospital mortality similar in anemic and nonanemic pts	Poor prognosis even in early-stage HF	
Berry et al,[2] 2016	13,295 pts (form MAGGIC data set)	Hb g/dL	Increased mortality, especially in older pts with high degree of comorbidity. Anemia alone was able to better stratify pts with HFpEF in lower and higher risk	Worse prognosis in HFrEF and anemia, followed by HFpEF with anemia equal to HFrEF without anemia. Higher mortality among women with higher nonanemic Hb levels (worsened arterial stiffness, sex-specific condition)	
Cattadori et al,[3] 2017	3913 pts from the MECKI score research group	Hb (very low/l ow/normal/ high in men and women) Multiparametric approach with CPET	At 5-y follow-up, pts with very low Hb had a reduction of survival compared with the other groups	Poor prognosis	

Study	Patients	Measure	Findings	
Abebe et al,[1] 2017	370 in-hospital pts (64.59% women)	Hb g/dL	Risk marker but not an independent predictor of mortality	Worse survival status
Tymińska et al,[10] 2017	1394 Caucasian pts hospitalized for HF	Hb g/dL	Mild to moderate anemia seems more a marker of older age, worse clinical condition, and a higher comorbidity burden, rather than an independent risk factor in HF	
Kajimoto et al,[6] 2017	4842 pts enrolled in the AHF Syndromes registry	Hb g/dL; Men and women with HFpEF or HFrEF	There was no adverse influence of anemia in men with HFpEF, whereas anemia was an independent predictor of all-cause death in men with HFrEF. Anemia was an independent predictor of all-cause death in women with HFpEF but not in women with HFrEF	In AHF patients, marked differences between men and women with respect to the association of anemia and LVEF with survival
Waldum et al,[12] 2012	4144 pts with HF, 21 clinics in Norway	Hb g/dL	Baseline anemia was not an independent predictor of all-cause mortality in outpatients with HF and severe renal dysfunction or advanced heart disease	Sustained anemia after HF treatment optimization might imply a worse prognosis independently of renal function and NYHA class
Kyriakou M. et al,[7] 2016	26 studies	Hb g/dL	Worse prognosis in HF patients with anemia. Nevertheless, the available data did not allow the extraction of a conclusion in which an exact Hb-level anemia becomes a negative predictor of prognosis	

Abbreviations: EF, ejection fraction; HFrEF, heart failure with reduced ejection fraction; pts, patients.

Table 2
Most common causes of anemia in patients with chronic heart failure

Cause	Mechanisms
Reduced iron absorption	• Reduced gut expression of hepcidin and ferroportin • Gut edema
Increased blood loss	• Bleeding (antiplatelet/ anticoagulant drugs, gastritis/ulcers) • Frequent blood tests (medical monitoring)
Bone marrow underproduction	• Cytokines production due to chronic inflammatory activation • Concomitant hematologic diseases
Renal function impairment	• RAAS system activation, sodium retention, and hemodilution • Reduced production of EPO • Proteinuria (loss of transferrin and erythropoietin) • ACEi high dosage treatments

Abbreviations: ACEi, angiotensin converting enzyme inhibitors; RAAS, renin-angiotensin-aldosterone system.

causes bone marrow blood cells underproduction and renin-angiotensin-aldosterone system activation, causing sodium and water retention with consequent hemodilution. Furthermore, renal insufficiency frequently affects patients with HF (partly because of vasoconstriction and renal ischemia) and entails not only reduced erythropoietin (EPO) production but also loss of EPO and transferrin due to the coexistence of proteinuria; in addition, angiotensin converting enzyme inhibitor treatment, especially at high dosage, can influence renal EPO production and bone marrow response to it.[13,15–18] Eventually, antiplatelet agents or anticoagulants can contribute to the presence of anemia and can cause blood loss.

Focus on Exercise Capacity in Heart Failure

Anemia is per se associated with impaired exercise performance and functional capacity, the Hb content playing a crucial and well-described role in determining the peak oxygen uptake (VO_{2peak}) value.[19] Agostoni and colleagues,[19] in a large cohort of patients with heart failure with reduced ejection fraction (HFrEF), showed that each gram of Hb accounts, on average, for a 0.97 mL/min/kg change in VO_{2peak}.[19] A few studies showed that, when anemia is treated, VO_{2peak} increases by a similar amount for each gram of Hb increase.[19] In such a context, some background of basic physiology might be useful. Practically, given that each Hb gram binds 1.34 mL of O_2 at 100% saturation and considering an expected mean O_2 extraction rate around 70% at peak exercise, each Hb gram should provide 1 mL of O_2. Thus, by multiplying 1 mL of O_2 by the CO (expressed in deciliters), one could obtain the amount of VO_{2peak} reduction due to the loss of 1 g/dL of Hb. For example, if peak exercise cardiac output is 7.0 L/min (=70 dL/min), and Hb is 10 g/dL, the amount of VO_{2peak} lacking due to anemia is 15 (normal Hb) − 10 (observed Hb) × 70 = 350 mL/min. Obviously, the abovementioned analysis is true only considering arterial O_2 saturation normal (ie, absence of cardiac shunt) and performing the exercise at sea level. Besides, it undoubtedly impacts VO_{2peak}, and low Hb content could impact also on ventilation-derived variables. Particularly, a recent subanalysis score, Metabolic Exercise and Cardiac and Kidney Indexes (MECKI score), focused on the possible effect of different Hb classes on the other 5 predictors.[20] Although the prognostic role of 4 of them has been confirmed, the ventilation versus carbon dioxide production (VE/VCO$_2$ slope) lost its prognostic power in severe anemic HF patients (Hb <11 g/dL) where its value was in any case the highest value. The physiology behind this observation is far to be elucidated even if it is supposed a role of the lactic acid–mediated chemoreceptor activation.[21]

Prognostic Significance in Heart Failure

Anemia is both a marker of HF severity and a predictor of poor prognosis in HF patients, as shown by several pieces of evidence, starting from the original studies of Silverberg and colleagues[17,18] until the most recent large multicenter studies. Berry and colleagues,[2] using the MAGGIC data set, which included 13,295 HF patients, showed that anemic HF patients were older, with a higher incidence of ischemic cause and with a more advanced HF class than the nonanemic counterpart. The MAGGIC data set analysis identified anemia as an independent predictor of adverse outcome in both heart failure with preserved ejection fraction (HFpEF) and HFrEF. Further support of its powerful prognostic role comes from the Metabolic Exercise Cardiac and Kidney Indexes (MECKI) study, including 2716 HFrEF patients in whom a score has been built and validated considering several cardiopulmonary exercise test (CPET), clinical, laboratory, and echocardiographic parameters. Again, the study identified the Hb as 1 of the 6 independent predictors of total and cardiovascular mortality, the others being VO_{2peak}, VE/VCO_2 slope, left ventricular ejection fraction (LVEF), renal function, and sodium.[20] Furthermore, a most recent MECKI score dataset analysis, including more than 6000 HFrEF patients with an average follow-up greater than 3 years, confirmed the datum.[3] Eventually, similar results were reported in a large meta-analysis,[7] whereby anemic HF patients showed the worse outcome. Interestingly, besides the presence of anemia per se, anemia kinetic seems also to have a strong impact both in chronic and in acute heart failure (AHF) patients. Indeed, a Norwegian-population study[12] suggested that only sustained anemia after HF-treatment optimization, but not the Hb baseline values, independently predicted the HF outcome. Supporting the importance of the Hb kinetic, in a large population of ambulatory HF patients, Diez-Lopez and colleagues[4] showed that anemia was an independent predictor of all-cause mortality, but the impact was more pronounced in the case of persistent and new-onset anemia. Similarly, in an AHF cohort, van der Meer and colleagues[11] showed that the in-hospital increase of Hb level predicted a better 180-day survival. Another recent study,[5] evaluating the in-hospital mortality in 165 hospitalized AHF patients, found Hb but not LVEF as an independent predictor. Interestingly, the same study identified also the red blood cell distribution width (RDW), an index of red blood cell inhomogeneity frequently available but rarely considered, significantly related to the survival. Overlapping observations on a possible RDW utility were reported by Tseliou and colleagues[9] on recently decompensated HF patients in whom it has been shown as a predictor of adverse outcome independently of the presence of an anemic status.

The administration of EPO-stimulating agents in disease settings closely associated with anemia has been evaluated in several studies. Recently, van der Meer and colleagues,[22] in the RED-HF study in HF patients, found that a poor response to darbepoetin alfa was associated with worse outcomes in HF patients with anemia. Another recent study[23] showed that a combined therapy in HF patients with anemia (methoxy polyethylene glycol-epoetin β and iron supplementation) improved overall physical condition, reduced HF symptoms and hospitalization frequency, as well as demonstrated a tendency to a general mortality reduction. Supporting the latter

study, another article[24] demonstrated that in HF the production of EPO is impaired as well as its capacity to induce an effective response, with a high degree of interpersonal variability. Particularly, the cited study showed that the EPO expression levels were elevated in HF patients, and HF patients with anemia have a positive correlation between the severity of HF and the anemic status degree.

IRON DEFICIENCY
Preliminary Overview on Iron Metabolism

Iron is probably the most important micronutrient for physiologic cellular function, playing various roles, energy metabolism, cell signaling, gene expression, and cell growth/differentiation.[25–30] In healthy humans, the total body iron amounts to nearly 3000 to 4000 mg, with a significant iron reserve stored in hepatocytes (1000 mg) as well as in macrophages of the reticuloendothelial system (600 mg). However, the greatest part of iron constitutes the so-called functional pool, where about 1800 mg is contained in the Hb of mature red blood cell, 300 mg in erythropoietic precursors in bone marrow, and 400 mg in myoglobin and different enzymes. Because the human body is not able to excrete excess iron, a tightly regulated system for iron homeostasis maintains the optimal balance between adequate dietary iron absorption and iron loss. Indeed, starting from about 10 mg of daily-ingested iron, only 2 mg is effectively absorbed by the gastrointestinal tract. Specifically, dietary iron is reduced to Fe^{2+} by duodenal cytochrome B in the lumen of the duodenum and proximal jejunum, and then it enters into the enterocyte thanks to the divalent metal transporter-1. Thereafter, iron passes into the circulation throughout ferroportin, is quickly oxidized to Fe^{3+}, and then is bound to transferrin. Eventually, the transferrin-iron complex is picked up by several target cells expressing transferrin receptor 1, including those of the liver, spleen, and bone marrow, where it is stored as ferritin.[31–34] The extracellular iron homeostasis is primarily regulated by the liver-derived peptide hormone hepcidin, whereas the intracellular one is dependent on autonomous mechanisms.[35,36] Briefly, in response to an iron overload condition or to an inflammatory state, hepcidin acts by binding and degrading ferroportin, thus inhibiting the iron transition to the circulation and leading to iron accumulation within enterocytes and excretion via shedding of the intestinal cells. Furthermore, because ferroportin is also present in the reticuloendothelial system, hepcidin leads to iron sequestration, and it reduces its availability. Noteworthy, hepcidin levels decrease in iron deficiency (ID) conditions in order to favor an increased iron absorption through the ferroportin activity[26,35–37] (**Fig. 1**).

Iron Deficiency: Definition, Prevalence, and Underlying Mechanisms in Heart Failure

Although ferritin is an intracellular storage molecule, a small amount can be measured in the bloodstream, and, especially in stable HF patients, serum ferritin has been shown to significantly correlate with overall iron stores measured by bone marrow aspirate.[38,39] Although the normal range for serum ferritin is 15 to 30 μg/L, ferritin is also an acute-phase protein, and therefore, it could increase during inflammatory states. Accordingly, both the European Society of Cardiology (ESC) and the American Heart Association (AHA) HF guidelines identified a serum ferritin less than 100 μg/L as the most accurate cutoff value to diagnose a state whereby there is truly insufficient iron ("absolute ID").[40–42] Conversely, in the case of a serum ferritin within 100 to 300 μg/L with a transferrin saturation (TSAT) of less than 20%, there is a condition whereby the available iron stores are preserved but cannot be transported from the intracellular compartment to the circulation ("functional ID").[26,35,37,42] Of note, differently from serum ferritin, TSAT is almost not affected by a possible concomitant inflammatory state.

ID has now emerged as an important comorbidity of HF,[43] the burdening prevalence of this condition being 30% to 50% of the overall HF patients[44,45] and even 70% to 80% in AHF.[46] Nonetheless, the diagnosis and correction of ID remain largely unrecognized in the cardiology community, despite the existence of relatively easy and inexpensive diagnostic tools and treatments. The ID pathophysiology in HF patients is undoubtedly multifactorial (**Table 3**). Indeed, besides a possible gastrointestinal ulceration or malignancy, there may be simple factors, such as blood loss due to antiplatelet or anticoagulant therapy, leading to iron loss. Similarly, poor absorption due to gut interstitial edema, possibly enhanced by a reduction in appetite from chronic illness, may lead to a reduction in iron body concentration. In addition, the chronic inflammatory state associated with HF leads to increased levels of proinflammatory cytokines, such as interleukin-6, which in turn induces the synthesis of hepcidin and hence a reduction in ferroportin expression

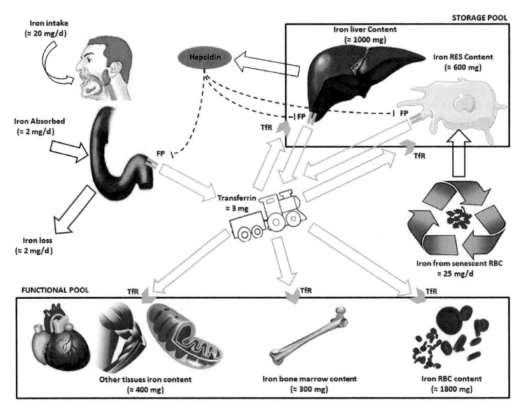

Fig. 1. Simplified diagram resembling the normal iron metabolism. See text for in-depth explanation. FP, ferroportin; RBC, red blood cell; RES, reticuloendothelial system; TfR, transferrin receptor.

Table 3
Most common causes of iron deficiency in patients with chronic heart failure

Cause	Mechanisms
Reduced iron intake	• Reduced appetite (chronic illness) • Low-protein diet (concomitant renal disease)
Reduced iron absorption	• Gut interstitial edema (mucosa congestion) • Impaired gut motility (concomitant dysautonomic disorders) • Impaired iron transporter expression at duodenum level (inflammation)
Increased iron loss	• Bleeding (antiplatelet/ anticoagulant drugs, gastritis/ulcers) • Enhanced iron storage consumption (chronic bleeding, concomitant therapy with erythropoiesis-stimulating agents) • Frequent blood tests (medical monitoring) • Malignancy
Impaired iron release	• Iron sequestration into the reticuloendothelial system (inflammation)

with a decrease in iron transition into the circulation as well as in its sequestration in the macrophages of the reticuloendothelial system. Intriguingly, a paradoxic behavior of this peptide has been observed in HF patients, with the higher hepcidin levels in the earlier rather than in the most advanced phases. The abovementioned phenomenon, It is still far from being understood, may be partly due to a usual concomitant EPO therapy in the worse HF stages, as well as to an overall reduction of liver activity.[26,35,37,47]

Iron Deficiency: Focus on Functional Capacity in Heart Failure

Iron plays a crucial role in O_2 transport (as a component of Hb), storage (as a component of myoglobin), and oxidative metabolism in muscle tissue (as a component of oxidative enzymes and respiratory chain proteins). A preserved iron metabolism is particularly important for cells characterized by intensive metabolism and high energy demand, such as exercising skeletal myocytes and cardiomyocytes.[27,32,48–50] In patients with HF, the presence of ID, irrespective of Hb levels,

has been associated with a reduced VO_{2peak} and an increased VE/VCO_2 slope as compared with subjects without ID.[25] However, the mechanism by which ID results in limited exercise capacity is multifactorial, but it remains elusive. Indeed, ID could affect both components of the Fick equation (CO and arterovenous difference), thereby resulting in a blunted VO_{2peak}. Otherwise, to date, there are only a few studies demonstrating that the correction of ID in HF patients, regardless of the presence of anemia, may favorably affect clinical status, including an improvement in exercise capacity.[51–54] Two large randomized, double-blind, placebo-controlled clinical trials, the FAIR-HF and CONFIRM-HF trials, have demonstrated that the intravenous (IV) supplementation of iron by ferric carboxymaltose in patients with HF and ID increases the distance of the 6-minute walk test (6-MWT) and improves functional capacity (New York Heart Association [NYHA] class) and overall quality of life in both anemic and nonanemic subjects.[53,55–58] A randomized controlled trial, FERRIC-HF, demonstrated that IV iron loading improved exercise capacity and symptoms in anemic and nonanemic patients with symptomatic HF and ID. The investigators demonstrated a significant improvement in maximal exercise capacity as quantified by VO_{2peak} (mL/min/kg) and trends toward an increase in absolute VO_{2peak} and exercise duration.[52]

Iron Deficiency: Prognostic Significance in Heart Failure

Oral iron replacement therapy, although relatively inexpensive and widely used, showed a great concern in its limited tolerability and, contextually, its low gastrointestinal absorption, particularly when gastrointestinal absorption has been hampered, as in chronic disease. Indeed, given that a dose of iron around 1000 mg is necessary to achieve a full iron repletion in HF patients with ID, and that the rate of iron bioavailability from a therapeutic dose of 200 mg oral ferrous sulfate (the usual oral iron formulation) is nearly 10%, the best-case scenario would be a truly absorbed iron dose of 20 mg per day, thus requiring nearly 2 months to correct the ID condition. However, it is well known that the best-case scenario is far from being the real-life scenario, where HF patients tolerate no more than a half dose of oral iron and show a significant impairment in the mechanisms needed to absorb iron and to favor its transition to the bloodstream. Furthermore, as previously mentioned, there are frequent side effects, such as constipation, diarrhea, and dyspepsia, which are predominantly related to

Table 4
Preparations, dosages, and administration of intravenous iron complexes

Preparations	Dosages[a]	Administration
Iron carboxymaltose (ie, Ferinject)	• 15 mg/kg (up to 1000 mg once per week) • Up to 200 mg/day (3 times per week)	IV infusion with 2 mg/mL iron concentration (in NaCl 0.9%) IV bolus (at least in 10 min)
Iron hydroxide sucrose (ie, Venofer)	• Up to 300 mg/day (3 times per week, 48-h intervals)	Slow (at least in 1.5 h) IV infusion (diluted in 100 mL of NaCl 0.9%)
Iron hydroxide dextran (ie, Ferrisat)	• Up to 20 mg/kg/day (3 times per week, 48-h intervals)	Slow (at least in 50 min) IV infusion (in 100 mL of NaCl 0.9% or glucose 5%)

[a] Total iron deficit could be calculated according to the Ganzoni formula[68]: weight, kg [a] (target Hb, g/dL – actual Hb, g/dL) × 2.4 + 500 (or 15 × weight, kg if weight <35 kg).

the oxidative damage of the mucosal boundary.[59] All of this may explain why all randomized trials exploring the possible efficacy of oral iron therapy failed to demonstrate any effect on quality of life or on functional capacity and, even on Hb, serum ferritin, and TSAT levels.[60–63] Furthermore, data from the IRON-HF trial (iron supplementation in HF patients with anemia), a study designed to compare the effect of oral versus IV iron therapy on exercise capacity, showed a clinically relevant difference in VO_{2peak} values (nearly 4 mL/kg/min) in the IV-treated arm.[64] Eventually, also following the overall negative results emerged from the recent IRONOUT study (Iron Repletion effects ON Oxygen UpTake in Heart Failure),[65] the oral iron supplementation therapy should be avoided in HF patients with ID. Differently from oral supplementation, the IV iron therapy avoids the gastrointestinal tract, thus significantly improving iron levels in the circulation and its availability for the target tissues. Besides several small studies involving less than 50 patients,[51,52,54,66] there is growing evidence from several randomized, placebo-controlled studies strongly supporting IV iron administration (**Table 4**), a beneficial therapeutic strategy to be adopted in HF patients with ID. The FAIR-HF study (Ferinject assessment in patients with ID and HF), conducted in 459 patients with HFrEF and ID, showed an improvement in quality of life, NYHA class, and 6-MWT in the treated arm.[53] Similarly, the CONFIRM-HF trial, on 304 HF patients, reported significant improvements in the same endpoint but also in time to first hospitalization.[55] Recently, the EFFECT-HF trial (Effect of Ferric Carboxymaltose on Exercise Capacity in Patients with Chronic Heart Failure and Iron Deficiency), on 172 HF patients, also suggested a slight improvement in a more objective functional parameter, such as VO_{2peak}, with respect to 6-MWT.[67] The weight of evidence from these large randomized trials has led the

last 2017-AHA (class IIB) and the 2016-ESC (class IIA) guidelines to recommend IV iron replacement therapy in the HF patients who meet the ID criteria.[40,41]

REFERENCES

1. Abebe TB, Gebreyohannes EA, Bhagavathula AS, et al. Anemia in severe heart failure patients: does it predict prognosis? BMC Cardiovasc Disord 2017;17(1):248.
2. Berry C, Poppe KK, Gamble GD, et al. Prognostic significance of anaemia in patients with heart failure with preserved and reduced ejection fraction: results from the MAGGIC individual patient data meta-analysis. QJM 2016;109(6):377–82.
3. Cattadori G, Agostoni P, Corra U, et al. Heart failure and anemia: effects on prognostic variables. Eur J Intern Med 2017;37:56–63.
4. Diez-Lopez C, Lupon J, de Antonio M, et al. Hemoglobin kinetics and long-term prognosis in heart failure. Rev Esp Cardiol (Engl Ed) 2016;69(9):820–6.
5. Dvornik S, Zaninovic Jurjevic T, Jurjevic N, et al. Prognostic factors for in-hospital mortality of patients hospitalized for acutely decompensated heart failure. Acta Clin Belg 2018;73(3):199–206.
6. Kajimoto K, Minami Y, Sato N, et al. Gender differences in anemia and survival in patients hospitalized for acute decompensated heart failure with preserved or reduced ejection fraction. Am J Cardiol 2017;120(3):435–42.
7. Kyriakou M, Kiff PF. Prognosis of the comorbid heart failure and anemia: a systematic review and meta-analysis. Clin Trials Regul Sci Cardiol 2016;16:12–21.
8. Migone de Amicis M, Chivite D, Corbella X, et al. Anemia is a mortality prognostic factor in patients initially hospitalized for acute heart failure. Intern Emerg Med 2017;12(6):749–56.
9. Tseliou E, Terrovitis JV, Kaldara EE, et al. Red blood cell distribution width is a significant prognostic

marker in advanced heart failure, independent of hemoglobin levels. Hellenic J Cardiol 2014;55(6): 457–61.

10. Tymińska A, Kaplon-Cieslicka A, Ozieranski K, et al. Anemia at hospital admission and its relation to outcomes in patients with heart failure (from the Polish Cohort of 2 European Society of Cardiology Heart Failure Registries). Am J Cardiol 2017;119(12): 2021–9.

11. van der Meer P, Postmus D, Ponikowski P, et al. The predictive value of short-term changes in hemoglobin concentration in patients presenting with acute decompensated heart failure. J Am Coll Cardiol 2013;61(19):1973–81.

12. Waldum B, Westheim AS, Sandvik L, et al. Baseline anemia is not a predictor of all-cause mortality in outpatients with advanced heart failure or severe renal dysfunction. Results from the Norwegian Heart Failure Registry. J Am Coll Cardiol 2012;59(4): 371–8.

13. Lupon J, Urrutia A, Gonzalez B, et al. [Prognostic significance of hemoglobin levels in patients with heart failure]. Rev Esp Cardiol 2005;58(1): 48–53.

14. Solomakhina NI, Nakhodnova ES, Belenkov YN. Anemia of chronic disease and iron deficiency anemia: comparative characteristics of ferrokinetic parameters and their relationship with inflammation in late middle-aged and elderly patients with CHF. Kardiologiia 2018;58(S8):58–64 [in Russian].

15. Hillege HL, Nitsch D, Pfeffer MA, et al. Renal function as a predictor of outcome in a broad spectrum of patients with heart failure. Circulation 2006; 113(5):671–8.

16. Go AS, Chertow GM, Fan D, et al. Chronic kidney disease and the risks of death, cardiovascular events, and hospitalization. N Engl J Med 2004; 351(13):1296–305.

17. Silverberg DS, Wexler D, Iaina A. The importance of anemia and its correction in the management of severe congestive heart failure. Eur J Heart Fail 2002; 4(6):681–6.

18. Silverberg DS, Wexler D, Sheps D, et al. The effect of correction of mild anemia in severe, resistant congestive heart failure using subcutaneous erythropoietin and intravenous iron: a randomized controlled study. J Am Coll Cardiol 2001;37(7): 1775–80.

19. Agostoni P, Salvioni E, Debenedetti C, et al. Relationship of resting hemoglobin concentration to peak oxygen uptake in heart failure patients. Am J Hematol 2010;85(6):414–7.

20. Agostoni P, Corra U, Cattadori G, et al. Metabolic exercise test data combined with cardiac and kidney indexes, the MECKI score: a multiparametric approach to heart failure prognosis. Int J Cardiol 2013;167(6):2710–8.

21. Chang AJ, Ortega FE, Riegler J, et al. Oxygen regulation of breathing through an olfactory receptor activated by lactate. Nature 2015;527(7577): 240–4.

22. van der Meer P, Grote Beverborg N, Pfeffer MA, et al. Hyporesponsiveness to Darbepoetin Alfa in patients with heart failure and anemia in the RED-HF study (reduction of events by darbepoetin alfa in heart failure): clinical and prognostic associations. Circ Heart Fail 2018;11(2): e004431.

23. Zahidova KK. Indexes of the erythropoietin level in the blood plasma of chronic heart failure patients with anemia. J Basic Clin Physiol Pharmacol 2018; 29(1):11–7.

24. Montero D, Haider T, Flammer AJ. Erythropoietin response to anaemia in heart failure. Eur J Prev Cardiol 2018;26(1):7–17.

25. Jankowska EA, Rozentryt P, Witkowska A, et al. Iron deficiency predicts impaired exercise capacity in patients with systolic chronic heart failure. J Card Fail 2011;17(11):899–906.

26. Musallam KM, Taher AT. Iron deficiency beyond erythropoiesis: should we be concerned? Curr Med Res Opin 2018;34(1):81–93.

27. Cairo G, Bernuzzi F, Recalcati S. A precious metal: iron, an essential nutrient for all cells. Genes Nutr 2006;1(1):25–39.

28. Ajioka RS, Phillips JD, Kushner JP. Biosynthesis of heme in mammals. Biochim Biophys Acta 2006; 1763(7):723–36.

29. Koskenkorva-Frank TS, Weiss G, Koppenol WH, et al. The complex interplay of iron metabolism, reactive oxygen species, and reactive nitrogen species: insights into the potential of various iron therapies to induce oxidative and nitrosative stress. Free Radic Biol Med 2013;65:1174–94.

30. Lill R, Hoffmann B, Molik S, et al. The role of mitochondria in cellular iron-sulfur protein biogenesis and iron metabolism. Biochim Biophys Acta 2012; 1823(9):1491–508.

31. Andrews NC. Disorders of iron metabolism. N Engl J Med 1999;341(26):1986–95.

32. Dunn LL, Suryo Rahmanto Y, Richardson DR. Iron uptake and metabolism in the new millennium. Trends Cell Biol 2007;17(2):93–100.

33. De Domenico I, McVey Ward D, Kaplan J. Regulation of iron acquisition and storage: consequences for iron-linked disorders. Nat Rev Mol Cell Biol 2008;9(1):72–81.

34. Gkouvatsos K, Papanikolaou G, Pantopoulos K. Regulation of iron transport and the role of transferrin. Biochim Biophys Acta 2012;1820(3): 188–202.

35. Anand IS, Gupta P. Anemia and iron deficiency in heart failure: current concepts and emerging therapies. Circulation 2018;138(1):80–98.

36. Ganz T. Hepcidin, a key regulator of iron metabolism and mediator of anemia of inflammation. Blood 2003;102(3):783–8.

37. Cohen-Solal A, Leclercq C, Deray G, et al. Iron deficiency: an emerging therapeutic target in heart failure. Heart 2014;100(18):1414–20.

38. Coenen JL, van Dieijen-Visser MP, van Pelt J, et al. Measurements of serum ferritin used to predict concentrations of iron in bone marrow in anemia of chronic disease. Clin Chem 1991; 37(4):560–3.

39. Cappellini MD, Comin-Colet J, de Francisco A, et al. Iron deficiency across chronic inflammatory conditions: international expert opinion on definition, diagnosis, and management. Am J Hematol 2017; 92(10):1068–78.

40. Ponikowski P, Voors AA, Anker SD, et al. 2016 ESC guidelines for the diagnosis and treatment of acute and chronic heart failure: the task force for the diagnosis and treatment of acute and chronic heart failure of the European Society of Cardiology (ESC). Developed with the special contribution of the Heart Failure Association (HFA) of the ESC. Eur J Heart Fail 2016;18(8):891–975.

41. Yancy CW, Jessup M, Bozkurt B, et al. 2017 ACC/ AHA/HFSA focused update of the 2013 ACCF/AHA guideline for the management of heart failure: a report of the American College of Cardiology/American Heart Association task force on clinical practice guidelines and the Heart Failure Society of America. J Am Coll Cardiol 2017;70(6):776–803.

42. Grote Beverborg N, Klip IT, Meijers WC, et al. Definition of iron deficiency based on the gold standard of bone marrow iron staining in heart failure patients. Circ Heart Fail 2018;11(2):e004519.

43. Jankowska EA, Malyszko J, Ardehali H, et al. Iron status in patients with chronic heart failure. Eur Heart J 2013;34(11):827–34.

44. von Haehling S, Jankowska EA, van Veldhuisen DJ, et al. Iron deficiency and cardiovascular disease. Nat Rev Cardiol 2015;12(11):659–69.

45. Klip IT, Comin-Colet J, Voors AA, et al. Iron deficiency in chronic heart failure: an international pooled analysis. Am Heart J 2013;165(4):575–582 e573.

46. Cohen-Solal A, Damy T, Terbah M, et al. High prevalence of iron deficiency in patients with acute decompensated heart failure. Eur J Heart Fail 2014; 16(9):984–91.

47. Leszek P, Sochanowicz B, Szperl M, et al. Myocardial iron homeostasis in advanced chronic heart failure patients. Int J Cardiol 2012;159(1):47–52.

48. Anderson GJ, Vulpe CD. Mammalian iron transport. Cell Mol Life Sci 2009;66(20):3241–61.

49. Munoz M, Villar I, Garcia-Erce JA. An update on iron physiology. World J Gastroenterol 2009;15(37): 4617–26.

50. Beard JL. Iron biology in immune function, muscle metabolism and neuronal functioning. J Nutr 2001; 131(2S-2):568S–79S [discussion: 580S].

51. Bolger AP, Bartlett FR, Penston HS, et al. Intravenous iron alone for the treatment of anemia in patients with chronic heart failure. J Am Coll Cardiol 2006;48(6):1225–7.

52. Okonko DO, Grzeslo A, Witkowski T, et al. Effect of intravenous iron sucrose on exercise tolerance in anemic and nonanemic patients with symptomatic chronic heart failure and iron deficiency FERRIC-HF: a randomized, controlled, observer-blinded trial. J Am Coll Cardiol 2008;51(2):103–12.

53. Anker SD, Comin Colet J, Filippatos G, et al. Ferric carboxymaltose in patients with heart failure and iron deficiency. N Engl J Med 2009;361(25): 2436–48.

54. Toblli JE, Lombrana A, Duarte P, et al. Intravenous iron reduces NT-pro-brain natriuretic peptide in anemic patients with chronic heart failure and renal insufficiency. J Am Coll Cardiol 2007;50(17): 1657–65.

55. Ponikowski P, van Veldhuisen DJ, Comin-Colet J, et al. Beneficial effects of long-term intravenous iron therapy with ferric carboxymaltose in patients with symptomatic heart failure and iron deficiency†. Eur Heart J 2015;36(11):657–68.

56. Filippatos G, Farmakis D, Colet JC, et al. Intravenous ferric carboxymaltose in iron-deficient chronic heart failure patients with and without anaemia: a subanalysis of the FAIR-HF trial. Eur J Heart Fail 2013;15(11):1267–76.

57. Van Craenenbroeck EM, Conraads VM, Greenlaw N, et al. The effect of intravenous ferric carboxymaltose on red cell distribution width: a subanalysis of the FAIR-HF study. Eur J Heart Fail 2013;15(7):756–62.

58. Ponikowski P, Filippatos G, Colet JC, et al. The impact of intravenous ferric carboxymaltose on renal function: an analysis of the FAIR-HF study. Eur J Heart Fail 2015;17(3):329–39.

59. Falkingham M, Abdelhamid A, Curtis P, et al. The effects of oral iron supplementation on cognition in older children and adults: a systematic review and meta-analysis. Nutr J 2010;9:4.

60. Palazzuoli A, Silverberg D, Iovine F, et al. Erythropoietin improves anemia exercise tolerance and renal function and reduces B-type natriuretic peptide and hospitalization in patients with heart failure and anemia. Am Heart J 2006;152(6):1096. e9-15.

61. van Veldhuisen DJ, Dickstein K, Cohen-Solal A, et al. Randomized, double-blind, placebo-controlled study to evaluate the effect of two dosing regimens of darbepoetin alfa in patients with heart failure and anaemia. Eur Heart J 2007;28(18):2208–16.

62. Ghali JK, Anand IS, Abraham WT, et al. Randomized double-blind trial of darbepoetin alfa in patients with

symptomatic heart failure and anemia. Circulation 2008;117(4):526–35.

63. Kourea K, Parissis JT, Farmakis D, et al. Effects of darbepoetin-alpha on quality of life and emotional stress in anemic patients with chronic heart failure. Eur J Cardiovasc Prev Rehabil 2008;15(3): 365–9.

64. Beck-da-Silva L, Piardi D, Soder S, et al. IRON-HF study: a randomized trial to assess the effects of iron in heart failure patients with anemia. Int J Cardiol 2013;168(4):3439–42.

65. Lewis GD, Malhotra R, Hernandez AF, et al. Effect of oral iron repletion on exercise capacity in patients with heart failure with reduced ejection fraction and iron deficiency: the IRONOUT HF randomized clinical trial. JAMA 2017;317(19):1958–66.

66. Usmanov RI, Zueva EB, Silverberg DS, et al. Intravenous iron without erythropoietin for the treatment of iron deficiency anemia in patients with moderate to severe congestive heart failure and chronic kidney insufficiency. J Nephrol 2008;21(2):236–42.

67. van Veldhuisen DJ, Ponikowski P, van der Meer P, et al. Effect of ferric carboxymaltose on exercise capacity in patients with chronic heart failure and iron deficiency. Circulation 2017;136(15):1374–83.

68. Ganzoni AM. Intravenous iron-dextran: therapeutic and experimental possibilities. Schweiz Med Wochenschr 1970;100:301–3.

Prognostic Value of Hormonal Abnormalities in Heart Failure Patients

Paola Gargiulo, MD, PhD[a],*, Stefania Paolillo, MD, PhD[a],
Francesca Ferrazzano, MD[b], Maria Prastaro, MD[b],
Lucia La Mura, MD[b], Anna Maria De Roberto, MD[b],
Gaetano Diana, MD[b], Simona Dell'Aversana, MD[b],
Cristina Contiello, MS[b], Maria Cristina Vozzella, MD[b],
Luca Bardi, MD[b], Fabio Marsico, MD[c]

KEYWORDS

- Chronic heart failure • Multiple hormone deficiency syndrome • Hormonal abnormalities

KEY POINTS

- Chronic heart failure (CHF) could be considered a multiple hormone deficiency syndrome.
- Reduced anabolic drive has relevant functional and prognostic implications.
- Anabolic deficiencies could provide additional utility for prognostic biomarker investigations as well as identify hormonal systems for targeted and personalized treatment strategies.

INTRODUCTION

Chronic heart failure (CHF) is a leading cause of mortality and morbidity in European countries. Approximately 1% to 2% of the adult population is affected by CHF in developed countries, with higher prevalence in the elderly (10% of men and 8% of women over the age of 60).[1] Despite remarkable progress in management of patients with CHF, mean survival in CHF is approximately 50% at 5 years, and up to 50% of patients are readmitted for CHF within 6 months of discharge.[2] Numerous clinical, imaging, and biohumoral parameters have been advocated as potential predictors of CHF prognosis, but they showed poor predictive power. As consequence, risk prediction remains challenging. For these reasons, researchers are looking for alternative models that could improve the understanding of the mechanisms underlining CHF progression.

The current model used to explain the pathophysiologic substrate and the progressive worsening in CHF is based on the hyperactivity of renin-angiotensin-aldosterone system and adrenergic pathway. Although enhanced activity of neurohormonal pathways is helpful to adapt the cardiac output to the needs of peripheral tissues and organs, it turns harmful in the long term and leads to pathologic left ventricular remodeling and disease CHF progression.[3] More than 20 years ago, large trials testing molecules inhibiting such hyperactivated pathways in CHF have demonstrated the clinical value of the neurohormonal model and determined the importance of routine use of several agents, including β-blockers, angiotensin-converting enzyme inhibitors, angiotensin receptor blockers, and aldosterone receptor antagonists. Although the neurohormonal traditional medical approach in the clinical setting has many advantages, it clearly

Disclosure: The authors have nothing to disclose.
[a] IRCCS SDN, Naples, Italy; [b] Department of Advanced Biomedical Sciences, Section of Cardiology, Federico II University of Naples, Naples, Italy; [c] Center for Congenital Heart Disease, University Hospital Inselspital, University of Bern, Bern, Switzerland
* Corresponding author. Via Pansini 5, Naples 80131, Italy.
E-mail address: paolagargiulo@hotmail.it

Heart Failure Clin 15 (2019) 371–375
https://doi.org/10.1016/j.hfc.2019.02.006
1551-7136/19/© 2019 Elsevier Inc. All rights reserved.

shows several pitfalls, as demonstrated by persistence of high rates of CHF mortality and hospitalization.

In the past decade, a growing body of evidence has led to the hypothesis that CHF is a multiple hormone deficiency syndrome (MHDS), characterized by a reduced anabolic drive that has relevant functional and prognostic implications.[4] The aim of this review is to summarize the evidence of reduced drive of main anabolic axes in CHF, emphasizing the prognostic role of multiple hormone deficiency in CHF.

ANDROGENS AND CHRONIC HEART FAILURE

The main androgens in the systemic circulation are testosterone, dihydrotestosterone, androstenedione, and dehydroepiandrosterone and its sulfate (DHEA-S). DHEA-S represents by far the most abundant androgen in the serum. Although DHEA-S is partially converted to testosterone, there is preliminary evidence about its direct actions, which are independent from androgen receptors, on several tissues, including endothelial cells and mediators of atherosclerosis.[5]

Approximately one-quarter of men with CHF display biochemical evidence of testosterone deficiency compared with age-matched healthy individuals.[6] In some studies, the reduction of testosterone levels is directly associated with functional measures of CHF, including distance at the 6-minute Walking test and peak oxygen consumption,[7] likely due to impaired skeletal muscle function. More importantly, androgens showed prognostic impact in CHF patients. In a study by Jankowska and colleagues,[6] baseline levels of total testosterone, DHEA-S, and insulinlike growth factor 1 (IGF-1) in male CHF patients have been assessed. Deficiency in each anabolic hormone was an independent marker of a poor prognosis, and multiple deficiencies identified groups with a higher mortality. Although androgen deficiency may indicate a poor outcome in patients with CHF and there are data linking low levels of testosterone to worse surrogate endpoints, there is no direct evidence that hypotestosteronemia alone may lead to a worse survival in CHF patients.

GROWTH HORMONE/INSULINLIKE GROWTH FACTOR 1 AND CHRONIC HEART FAILURE

In patients with CHF, the prognostic role of IGF-1 is controversial. Although few reports are not concordant, most studies found lower IGF-1 levels in patients with CHF compared with controls.[4] These results did not translate into a clear-cut evidence for IGF-1 as a strong predictor of mortality in CHF. Jankowska and colleagues[6] found that low IGF-1 was associated with higher mortality in CHF (in association with other anabolic deficiencies), whereas other studies were not congruent with this finding. An elevated growth hormone (GH/)IGF-1 ratio, but not IGF-1 alone, has shown to predict higher mortality,[8] whereas a recent Danish study addressing the role of IGF-1 as a predictor of CHF progression and all-cause mortality did not establish significant associations.[9] To address the predictive role of IGF-1 in CHF, Arcopinto and colleagues[10] prospectively studied a population of 207 consecutive patients with CHF, New York Heart Association (NYHA) classes I to III, with left ventricular (LV) ejection fraction of 40% or below. All patients underwent blood sample for circulating levels of IGF-1 and serum IGF binding protein-3 dosage, physical examination, and an echocardiographic study and cardiopulmonary exercise test. Patients were regularly followed-up in an outpatient clinic for a median period of 3.5 years (range 1–72 months). IGF-1 and IGF-1receptors levels were directly related to peak oxygen consumption (Vo_2) consumption ($r = .25$ and $r = .31$, respectively). No correlations were found between the hormones and LV volumes, LV ejection fraction, or N-terminal prohormone of brain natriuretic peptide (NT-proBNP). A tight, positive correlation between IGF-1mr and total IGF-1 levels also was found ($r = .68$; $p<0.0001$). Patients with lower IGF-1 showed significantly lower survival than those with higher values (log rank 13.8; p b .0001). In particular, death rates in patients with IGF-1 levels above or below a cutoff value derived from receiver operating curve analysis were 39.3% and 13.8%, respectively. The univariate Cox proportional hazards analysis found that higher NYHA class, diabetes mellitus (DM) presence, NT-proBNP levels, and renal function levels also were predictive of all-cause mortality in the population. Multivariate analysis, including the significant predictors in addition to IGF-1, indicated that IGF-1 maintained its predictive value and was significantly and independently associated with all-cause mortality (hazard ratio 2.46; 95% CI, 1.43–9.04; $P = .015$). Despite the small sample size and high dropout rate, this study for the first time reports that IGF-1 circulating levels are independent predictors of mortality in CHF. More recently, Arcopinto and colleagues[11] studied 130 CHF patients who underwent GH provocative test with GH-releasing hormone plus arginine. Accordingly with test results, authors categorized patients into GH deficiency (GHD) and GH sufficiency (GHS) GHD was detected in approximately 30% of CHF patients.

Compared with GHD, GHS patients showed smaller end-diastolic and end-systolic LV volumes, lower LV end-systolic wall stress, higher right ventricular performance, higher Vo_2, and increased ventilatory efficiency. After adjusting for clinical covariates (age, gender, tertiles of LV ejection fraction, IGF-1, peak Vo_2, minute ventilation [VE]/carbon dioxide output [Vco_2] slope, and NT-proBNP), logistic multivariate analysis showed that peak Vo_2, VE/Vco_2 slope, and NT-proBNP were significantly associated with GHD status. Finally, compared with GHS, GHD cohort showed higher all-cause mortality at median follow-up of 3.5 years (40% vs. 25%; $P<.001$, respectively), independent of age, gender, NT-proBNP, peak Vo_2, and LV ejection fraction. As a consequence, GHD should identify a subgroup of CHF patients characterized by impaired functional capacity, LV remodeling, neurohormonal activation, and poor prognosis. Future prospective trials, including the ongoing Trattamento Ormonale nello Scompenso Cardiaco (Hormone Therapy in Heart Failure) Registry,[12] will help delineate the impact of anabolic deficiencies, such as GHD, on CHF progression.

THYROID HORMONES AND CHRONIC HEART FAILURE

The well-known stimulating effects of thyroid hormones on contractile and relaxation LV properties and their role in the maintenance of a normal cardiac structure and function have represented an active field of interest for both cardiologists and endocrinologists. Subjects affected with subclinical hypothyroidism have a moderately increased risk of HF after a follow-up of 12 years.[13] Abnormal thyroid function in patients with symptomatic CHF is associated with a significantly increased risk for death, even after controlling for known mortality predictors.[14] In addition, it is recognized in approximately 20% to 30% of patients with CHF and without thyroid disease a characteristic defect in thyroid metabolism called, low T_3 syndrome, characterized by low levels of T_3 (likely due to impaired conversion of T_4 to T_3), with no significant alterations in T_4 and TSH. Iervasi and colleagues[15] documented increased all-cause mortality in cardiac patients with low T_3 levels. Since then, few studies have evaluated short-term replacement therapy with thyroid hormones (intravenous lev triiodothyronine) showing favorable hemodynamic effects, including enhanced resting cardiac output and reduced systemic vascular resistance as well as neuroendocrine deactivation.[16] No long-term studies are available. One problem is that T_3 has

a much shorter half-life than T_4 (approximately 1 day vs 7 days), and levothyroxine cannot be used because proper conversion to T_3 is the pathophysiologic defect in the low T_3 syndrome.

INSULIN RESISTANCE AND CHRONIC HEART FAILURE

Whole-body insulin resistance (IR) predicts CHF independently of other risk factors, and patients with CHF are predisposed to IR or overt DM.[17,18] In nondiabetic patients with CHF, IR shows high prevalence (up to 60%) and is associated with more aggressive CHF.[19] IR causes functional, metabolic, and structural alterations that ultimately generate myocardial damage and CHF progression. Perturbation in myocardial metabolism and energetics, caused by reduction of myocardial glucose uptake and increased free fatty acid myocardial uptake,[20] is a metabolic main mechanism involved in CHF progression.[19] In addition, the impaired expression of contractile proteins is responsible of depressed myofibrillar ATP activities as well as abnormalities of the sarcoplasmic reticular and sarcolemmal calcium transport processes, with consequent calcium overload and impaired diastolic performance.[21] Furthermore, microvascular and endothelial dysfunction, through repetitive ischemic insults, could contribute to CHF progression.[22,23] As recently reported, neurohormonal and sympathetic nervous systems activation[24,25] play a central role in prognosis worsening in HF patients with DM and IR. HF patients with DM or without DM but with IR show more impaired cardiac sympathetic innervation compared with nondiabetic and non-IR patients, indicating chronic adrenergic hyperactivity that correlates with hemoglobin A_{1c} levels and IR indices.[24,25] IR in CHF patients predisposes to poor survival.[26,27] However, overcoming of IR could represent an appealing, additive therapeutic target. Unfortunately, most available drugs that reduce IR in patients with type 2 DM also present with potential adverse effects in CHF (metformin and thiazolidinedione) for potential negative effect in CHF patients.

MULTIPLE HORMONE DEFICIENCY SYNDROME AND PROGNOSIS IN CHRONIC HEART FAILURE

As discussed previously, many studies demonstrated that not only does each component of MHDS (eg, GH/IGF-1 axes, thyroid hormones, androgens, and IR) have a high prevalence in HF but also hormonal defects have a negative impact on cardiovascular performance (**Table 1**). In 2006,

Table 1
Effect of hormonal abnormalities in chronic heart failure

Axis	Effect on Prognosis of Chronic Heart Failure Patients (Level of Evidence)	References
Androgens	(+)	6,7
IGF-1	(++)	4,8–10
GH	(+++)	11,12
Low T$_3$	(++)	13–16
IR	(++)	17–26
MHDS	(+++)	6,11,26

MHDS: for example, GH/IGF-1 axes, thyroid hormones, androgens, and IR.

Abbreviations: MHDS, multiple hormone deficiency syndrome; (+), questionable; (++), documented by powerful studies; and (+++), documented by powerful-long term studies.

Jankowska and colleagues[6] demonstrated that deficiency in each anabolic hormone was an independent marker of a poor prognosis, and multiple deficiencies identified groups with a higher mortality. Specifically, the 3-year survival rate was 83% in patients with no deficiencies, 74% in patients with 1 deficiency, 55% in patients with 2 deficiencies, and 27% in patients with deficiencies in all axes. More recently, Arcopinto and colleagues[11] demonstrated that in a population of approximately 200 stable chronic HF patients, fewer than a fifth presented with no signs of hormonal deficiency. Moreover, in patients with 2 or more deficiencies, cardiovascular performance was impaired, as demonstrated by a decreased ability for maximal oxygen uptake (and elevated levels of circulating NT-proBNP). Furthermore, the presence and number of deficiencies were related, with a poor prognosis for all-cause mortality.

These data are in line with those presented by Jankowska and colleagues,[6] reinforcing the relationship between the number of hormonal deficiencies and CHF outcomes. In addition, Arcopinto and colleagues[11] demonstrated that CHF has a heavy impact on age-related decline of anabolic drive. Specifically, CHF should attenuate DHEAS and IGF-1 decline, with a paradoxic inversion observed for testosterone. This could suggest MHDS has strong impact on young patients, with significant impact on quality of life. In 2016, a similar finding was demonstrated for the first time in patients with CHF with preserved ejection fraction (HFpEF).[26] Although fewer patients with HFpEF present reduced levels of MHDS compared with the CHF population with reduced ejection fraction, a remarkable prevalence of hormonal deficiency was documented. In particular, approximately 45% of the study population displayed 2 or more signs of hormone deficiency. The higher level of anabolic drive in CHFpEF, however, could further support the notion that CHFpEF should be considered distinct from heart failure with reduced ejection fraction. Also for CHFpEF, anabolic deficiencies could provide additional utility for prognostic biomarker investigations as well as identify hormonal systems for targeted and personalized treatment strategies.

Together, these data suggest that screening for MHDS should be performed routinely in patients diagnosed with CHF, due to the elevated prevalence of MHDS in HF and its impact on disease CHF progression and prognosis.

REFERENCES

1. Roger VL, Go AS, Lloyd-Jones DM, et al. Executive summary: heart disease and stroke statistics-2012 update: a report from the American Heart Association. Circulation 2012;125(1):188–97.
2. Laribi S, Aouba A, Nikolaou M, et al. Trends in death attributed to heart failure over the past two decades in Europe. Eur J Heart Fail 2012;14(3):234–9.
3. Mann DL, Bristow MR. Mechanisms and models in heart failure: the biomechanical model and beyond. Circulation 2005;111:2837–49.
4. Sacca L. Heart failure as a multiple hormonal deficiency syndrome. Circ Heart Fail 2009;2:151–6.
5. Komesaroff PA. Unravelling the enigma of dehydroepiandrosterone: moving forward step by step. Endocrinology 2008;149:886–8.
6. Jankowska EA, Biel B, Majda J, et al. Anabolic deficiency in men with chronic heart failure: prevalence and detrimental impact on survival. Circulation 2006;114:1829–37.
7. Pugh PJ, Jones RD, West JN, et al. Testosterone treatment for men with chronic heart failure. Heart 2004;90:446–7.
8. Petretta M, Colao A, Sardu C, et al. NT-proBNP, IGF-I and survival in patients with chronic heart fail-ure. Growth Horm IGF Res 2007;17:288–96.
9. Andreassen M, Kistorp C, Raymond I, et al. Plasma insulin-like growth factor I as predictor of progression and all cause mortality in chronic heart failure. Growth Horm IGF Res 2009;19:486–90.
10. Arcopinto M, Isgaard J, Marra AM, et al. IGF-1 predicts survival in chronic heart failure. Insights from the T.O.S.CA. (Trattamento Ormonale Nello Scompenso CArdiaco) registry. Int J Cardiol 2014; 176(3):1006–8.

11. Arcopinto M, Salzano A, Giallauria F, et al. Growth Hormone Deficiency Is Associated with Worse Cardiac Function, Physical Performance, and Outcome in Chronic Heart Failure: Insights from the T.O.S.CA. GHD Study. PLoS One 2017;12(1): e0170058.

12. Bossone E, Arcopinto M, Iacoviello M, et al. Multiple hormonal and metabolic deficiency syndrome in chronic heart failure: rationale, design, and demographic characteristics of the T.O.S.CA. Registry. Intern Emerg Med 2018;13(5):661–71.

13. Rodondi N, Bauer DC, Cappola AR, et al. Subclinical thyroid dysfunction, cardiac function, and the risk of heart failure. The Cardiovascular Health study. J Am Coll Cardiol 2008;52:1152–9.

14. Mitchell JE, Hellkamp AS, Mark DB, et al. Thyroid function in heart failure and impact on mortality. JACC Heart Fail 2013;1:48–55.

15. Iervasi G, Pingitore A, Landi P, et al. Low-T_3 syndrome: a strong prognostic predictor of death in patients with heart disease. Circulation 2003;107: 708–13.

16. Pingitore A, Galli E, Barison A, et al. Acute effects of triiodothyronine (T_3) replacement therapy in patients with chronic heart failure and low-T_3 syndrome: a randomized, placebo-controlled study. J Clin Endocrinol Metab 2008;93:1351–8.

17. Ingelsson E, Sundstrom J, Arnlov J, et al. Insulin resistance and risk of congestive heart fail- ure. JAMA 2005;294:334–41.

18. Gargiulo P, Perrone-Filardi P. Heart failure, whole-body insulin resistance and myocardial insulin resistance: An intriguing puzzle. J Nucl Cardiol 2018; 25(1):177–80.

19. Perrone-Filardi P, Paolillo S, Costanzo P, et al. The role of metabolic syndrome in heart failure. Eur Heart J 2015;36(39):2630–4.

20. Stanley WC, Lopaschuk GD, McCormack JG. Regulation of energy substrate metabolism in the diabetic heart. Cardiovasc Res 1997;34(1):25–33.

21. Dhalla NS, Liu X, Panagia V, et al. Subcellular remodeling and heart dysfunction in chronic diabetes. Cardiovasc Res 1998;40(2):239–47.

22. Marciano C, Galderisi M, Gargiulo P, et al. Effects of type 2 diabetes mellitus on coronary microvascular function and myocardial perfusion in patients without obstructive coronary artery disease. Eur J Nucl Med Mol Imaging 2012;39(7):1199–206.

23. Gargiulo P, Marciano C, Savarese G, et al. Endothelial dysfunction in type 2 diabetic patients with normal coronary arteries: a digital reactive hyperemia study. Int J Cardiol 2013;165(1):67–71.

24. Paolillo S, Rengo G, Pagano G, et al. Impact of diabetes on cardiac sympathetic innervation in patients with heart failure: a 123I meta-iodobenzylguanidine (123I MIBG) scintigraphic study. Diabetes Care 2013;36(8):2395–401.

25. Paolillo S, Rengo G, Pellegrino T, et al. Insulin resistance is associated with impaired cardiac sympathetic innervation in patients with heart failure. Eur Heart J Cardiovasc Imaging 2015;16(10):1148–53.

26. Doehner W, Rauchhaus M, Ponikowski P, et al. Impaired insulin sensitivity as an independent risk factor for mortality in patients with stable chronic heart failure. J Am Coll Cardiol 2005;46:1019–26.

27. Salzano A, Marra AM, Ferrara F, et al. Multiple hormone deficiency syndrome in heart failure with preserved ejection fraction. Int J Cardiol 2016;225:1–3.

Hormonal Replacement Therapy in Heart Failure
Focus on Growth Hormone and Testosterone

Andrea Salzano, MD, MRCP[a,b], Roberta D'Assante, PhD[c],
Mark Lander, MBBS, MRCP[d], Michele Arcopinto, MD[b,e],
Eduardo Bossone, MD, PhD[f], Toru Suzuki, MD, PhD[a],
Antonio Cittadini, MD[b,g,*]

KEYWORDS

- Heart failure • Hormones • Growth hormone • Testosterone • Cardiovascular disease
- Prognosis outcome • Therapy

KEY POINTS

- Heart failure can be considered as a multiple hormone deficiencies syndrome.
- Among hormone deficiencies, growth hormone deficit and testosterone deficit play a pivotal role.
- Growth hormone deficiency and testosterone deficiency are per se related to impaired cardiovascular performance and poor prognosis.
- The correction of growth hormone deficiency, as well as of testosterone deficiency (ie, hormonal replacement treatment), is safe and effective.

INTRODUCTION

To date, the mainstay of heart failure (HF) treatment is considered the counteraction of neurohormonal overactivation.[1] Indeed, according to the namesake pathophysiological model, even if the renin-angiotensin-aldosterone system together with the adrenergic system play a compensatory role in the early phases of the disease, they soon themselves become responsible for the progression of HF, triggering a vicious cycle of ever more deleterious increasing neurohormonal action.[2,3] Thus, the main target of HF therapy is to block this pattern using drugs such as angiotensin-converting enzyme (ACE) inhibitors, angiotensin receptor blockers, beta-blockers, mineral receptor antagonists, and the novel angiotensin receptor-neprilysin inhibitors. However, because of the activation of alternative escape pathways limiting the ability to completely prevent the natural progression of HF, the positive effects of these drugs are limited.

In this context, a dangerous link exists between hormones and cardiovascular system.[4–8] To date, growing evidence supports the concept

Disclosure Statement: Dr A. Salzano receives research grant support from Cardiopath, UniNA and Compagnia di San Paolo in the frame of Programme STAR.
[a] Department of Cardiovascular Sciences, NIHR Leicester Biomedical Research Centre, University of Leicester, Glenfield Hospital, Groby Road, Leicester LE3 9QP, UK; [b] Department of Translational Medical Sciences, Federico II University, Via Pansini 5, Naples 80138, Italy; [c] IRCCS SDN, Naples, Italy; [d] Department of Acute Medicine, University College London Hospitals NHS Foundation Trust, 235 Euston Road, London NW1 2BU, UK; [e] Emergency Department, A Cardarelli Hospital, Via Cardarelli 9, Naples 80131, Italy; [f] Cardiology Division, A Cardarelli Hospital, Via Cardarelli 9, Naples 80131, Italy; [g] Interdisciplinary Research Centre in Biomedical Materials (CRIB), Piazzale Tecchio 80, Naples 80125, Italy
* Corresponding author. Department of Translational Medical sciences, "Federico II" University–School of Medicine, Via Sergio Pansini 5, Napoli 80138, Italy.
E-mail addresses: antonio.cittadini@unina.it; cittadin@unina.it

Heart Failure Clin 15 (2019) 377–391
https://doi.org/10.1016/j.hfc.2019.02.007
1551-7136/19/

that hormonal deficiencies (HDs) in HF have a high prevalence and a strong impact on the disease, with a promising possible role of hormonal therapy.[9,10] In this intricate scenario, growth hormone deficiency (GHD) and testosterone deficiency (TD) seem to play a particularly critical role[11]. Most studies in the field demonstrated that patients affected by these disorders display a more aggressive phenotype of HF. However, the impact of multiple and concomitant HD (eg, growth hormone [GH] and insulin-like growth factor [IGF]-1, testosterone, insulin resistance [IR], thyroid) on adverse cardiovascular outcomes (eg, hospitalization and mortality rate) in HF is not completely elucidated, although a growing body of evidence suggests that treatment of these might have a role in HF.[12-15]

This article gives an overview of the current evidence regarding GHD and TD in HF and reviews the impact of their treatment in HF.

GROWTH HORMONE TREATMENT IN HEART FAILURE
Growth Hormone Deficiency in Heart Failure

The prevalence of GHD ranges from 32% to 53%.[16-19] The literature suggests that IGF-1 serum levels are decreased in HF subjects when compared with healthy subjects.[16,20-23] Of note, this finding is particularly evident in more advanced HF patients[24,25] or those with cachexia.[26,27]

Despite current guidelines suggesting insulin tolerance testing as the gold standard test for diagnosis of GHD in adults,[28-31] because hypoglycemia could be unsafe in the HF setting, alternative tests are often used instead. The GF–releasing hormone (GHRH) and arginine test could be considered the more convenient option.[16,32-35]

Several independent groups have demonstrated that GHD is per se related to impaired cardiovascular performance and increased peripheral vascular resistance, with a clear association between GHD severity, cardiac impairment,[36] and increased cardiovascular mortality.[37] Recently, combining stimulated pituitary responses with measures of the IGF-1 system in a cohort of HF subjects, Arcopinto and colleagues[22] demonstrated that GHD subjects displayed higher filling pressures with larger left ventricular (LV) volumes, and a more severe impairment of right ventricle systolic function in respect to non-GHD subjects. Further, a significantly lower peak oxygen consumption per unit time (Vo_2) and reduced ventilator efficiency have been demonstrated in the GHD group, resulting in impaired cardiopulmonary performance. Of note, patients with coexistent GHD

and chronic HF (CHF) display a higher risk of mortality compared with the GH-sufficient cohort (hazard ratio 2.11, $P = .021$). With regard to HF with preserved ejection fraction (HFpEF), it has been demonstrated that GHD is a common finding, although to a lower degree when compared with HF with reduced ejection fraction (HFrEF).[18]

In the acute setting, a relationship between GH status and outcome has been demonstrated.[38] In 537 acute HF subjects, GH levels were increased in all subjects who died or were readmitted to hospital within 1 year, regardless of their ejection fraction (EF). In this setting, GH levels were independently predictors of poor outcome in HFrEF but not in HFpEF. When added to the ADHERE multivariate model,[39] GH was able to ameliorate the net reclassification improvement, as well as when added to the acute decompensated heart failure national registry (ADHERE) model plus N-terminal pro (NT-proBNP). Despite some limitations (eg, the single GH measurement taken in nonfasted patients), for the first time GH activity has shown promise as a prognostic marker in the acute settings. To date, no data are available around the prevalence and role of GHD in acute HF.

Mechanisms of Growth Hormone Deficiency in Heart Failure

Local hypoperfusion of the hypothalamic-pituitary axis (with somatotopic cell death from mismatched arterial and venous flow)[16,40] alterations related to chronic disease (as well as in other several chronic wasting conditions characterized by liver congestion, inflammatory activation, and cytokine overexpression)[41] and/or effects of CHF therapy on the GH–IGF-1 axis[42,43] have been considered as the possible explanatory pathophysiological mechanism of the occurrence of GH–IGF-1 axis impairment in CHF. Current understanding suggests a multiple model in which the synergy and the interaction of these different molecular pathways with the concomitant pharmacologic action could explain the GH–IGF-1 axis alterations.[44,45]

Growth Hormone Treatment in Heart Failure

Data derived from animal models have shown several beneficial effects of GH on cardiac morphology and function, peripheral vascular resistance, and survival.[46-50] With regard to the pathophysiological mechanisms, it is well-recognized that GH therapy in myocardial infarction in the early stage improves LV function, mainly through a reduction of the pathologic LV remodeling.[51] However, results in the human CHF population remain inconsistent[52-68] when applied into

Table 1
Summary of studies on growth hormone treatment in heart failure

First Author (Year)	Sample Size	Gender	Mean Age (Years)	Baseline NYHA Class (Mean)	Growth Hormone Status	Growth Hormone Supplementation	Type of Trial	Trial Duration
Fazio et al,[52] 1996	7	Male (71) Female (29)	46	2.7 ± 0.2	NA	4 IU every other day SC	—	3 mo treatment and 3 mo after
Frustaci et al,[53] 1996	5	Male (25) Female (75)	28	NR	NA	4 IU daily IM	—	3 mo
Isgaard et al,[54] 1998	22	Male (64) Female (36)	60	3 ± 0.5	NA	0.1 IU/kg/wk for 1 wk, thereafter 0.25 IU/kg/wk	R, DB, PC	3 mo
Osterziel et al,[55,60] 1998	50	Male (86) Female (14)	54	2.3 ± 0.6	NA	0.5 IU or placebo daily, SC Dosage increased every second day by 0.5 IU until a final dose of 2 IU daily was reached	R, DB, PC	3 mo
Genth-Zotz et al,[56] 1999	7	Male	55	2.4 ± 0.5	NA	2 IU daily SC	—	3 mo treatment and 3 mo after
Jose et al, 1999[58]	6	NA	NR	3.4 ± 0.5	NA	2 IU every other day SC	—	6 mo treatment and 6 mo after
Spallarossa et al,[57] 1999	20	Male	62	2.7 ± 0.4	NA	0.0006 IU/kg daily SC Gradual increase until 0.02 IU/kg/daily	R, PC	6 mo
Smit et al,[59,64] 2001	19	Male (85) Female (15)	65	2.5 ± 0.7	NA	Start 0.5 IU daily SC Dosage increased to 1.0 IU/day after 2 wk and to 2.0 IU/day final dose	R, C	6 mo
Napoli et al,[61] 2002	16	Male (75) Female (25)	54	2.25 ± 0.4	NA	4 IU every other day SC	R, DB, PC	3 mo
Acevedo et al,[63] 2003	19	Male (90) Female (10)	57	3	NA	0.035 IU/Kg daily SC	R, DB, PC	2 mo
Adamopoulos et al,[62] 2003	12	Male (67) Female (33)	50	3	NA	4 IU every other day	R	3 mo treatment and 3 mo after
Fazio et al,[65] 2007	22	Male (69) Female (31)	55	2.45 ± 0.5	NA	4 IU every other day	R, DB, PC	3 mo
Cittadini et al,[19] 2009	56	Male (72) Female (28)	62	2.6 ± 0.7	GHD	0.012 mg/kg every other day	R, SB, C	6 mo
Cittadini et al,[74] 2013	31	Male (84) Female (16)	62	2.7 ± 0.1	GHD	0.012 mg/kg every other day	R, SB, C	48 mo

Abbreviations: C, controlled; DB, double-blind; IM, intramuscular; IU, international unit; NA, not assessed; NR, not reported; NYHA, New York Heart Association; PC, placebo-controlled; SB, single-blind.

clinical studies (**Table 1**). In the early 1990s, preliminary pilot studies verified the effects of GH treatment leading to positive results in CHF[52,53,56–58,61,63,65] as well as in other clinical settings.[69] However, when these results were tested in randomized controlled clinical trials,[54,55,60–63,65] previous encouraging results were not confirmed. Specifically, in a population of 50 CHF subjects, Osterziel and colleagues[55] demonstrated an increase in LV mass strongly related to serum IGF-1 changes but not to a clinical improvement in subjects with CHF. Of note, EF increased noticeably in subjects with the larger increases of IGF-1 during GH treatment.[60] Isgaard and colleagues,[54] as well as Acevedo and colleagues,[63] showed neutral effects of GH therapy in CHF subjects, although the latter demonstrated a positive relationship between the changes in Vo_2 and EF in the GH therapy group. In subjects with idiopathic dilated cardiomyopathy, a beneficial modulation of circulating cytokines and soluble adhesion molecules has been demonstrated by Adamopoulos and colleagues[62] in a randomized crossover trial, together with the positive effects of GH in contractile reserve and LV volumes. Marra and colleagues[70] confirmed the relationship between the cytokine network, cardiac performance, and survival in HF. Finally, in a double-blind, placebo randomized controlled trial, Fazio and colleagues[65] demonstrated that GH increased IGF-1 serum levels and improved New York Heart Association (NYHA) functional class and cardiopulmonary performance without affecting lung function parameters. None of these effects were observed in the placebo group.

Considering these results and with the aim of clarifying the overall effect of GH treatment in HF, Le Corvoisier and colleagues[12] performed a pooled meta-analysis of effects of GH therapy in CHF. In brief, sustained GH treatment improves cardiovascular parameters in HF (in particular, left ventricular ejection fraction [LVEF]) with a reduction in general vascular resistance. These changes were associated with a positive long-term modification in cardiac morphology, due to an increase in LV wall thickness and a reduction in LV diastolic diameters.[12] Tritos and Danias,[13] in different meta-analysis, demonstrated that GH treatment resulted in an improvement in systemic vascular resistance, an increase of cardiac output, LVEF, and NYHA class level, together with a significant improvement in exercise duration and in peak Vo_2. No effects were observed with regard to diastolic function. It is necessary to underline that there is a great inhomogeneity of data with regard to study duration, target dose, end-points, and the lack of assessment of GH status.[9] When

trials were separated in 2 groups according to the target dose of all clinical trials, Le Corvoisier and colleagues[12] demonstrated that a low GH dose affected only NYHA class and exercise duration, whereas a high GH dose positively affected ventricular morphology, cardiopulmonary performance, and clinical status. Subgroup analysis according to the median of IGF-1 increase showed that larger IGF-1 increases corresponded with a more significant effect size for LV morphology and cardiopulmonary performance. However, a neutral effect was observed in trials with smaller IGF-1 increases. Recently Brankovic and colleagues,[71–73] in a cohort of 263 CHF subjects from the Bio-SHiFT study, demonstrated that the temporal patterns of IGF binding proteins (IGFBPs), in particular IGFBP-1, IGFBP-2, and IGFBP-7, predict adverse clinical outcomes and could in part explain the nonresponsiveness of some patients to GH treatment, Taken all together, several findings from these meta-analyses can be considered and translated into clinical practice. First, before starting GH administration, a proven impairment of GH-IGF-1 status (eg, GHD) should be confirmed. Second, dose titration should be individualized. Third, GH therapy should not be administered in all patients with CHF but rather the subgroup of patients in which GH treatment is more effective (eg, mild to moderate CHF, considering the GH resistance state of the more advanced disease[27]).

In a randomized, single-blind controlled proof-of-concept trial, Cittadini and colleagues[19] were the first to assess the effects of GH therapy only in those patients suffering from GHD. In this study, subjects underwent a GHRH plus arginine provocative test with the aim of understanding GHD status; thus, only when GHD was diagnosed was GH treatment was started. After 6 months of GH replacement treatment, the investigators observed a decrease in circulating NT-proBNP levels and an improvement of LVEF (33 ± 2%–36 ± 2%, $P<.01$) and peak Vo_2 (12.9 ± 0.9–14.5 ± 1.0 mL/kg/min, $P<.005$), together with a better quality of life score and flow-mediated vasodilation. Because of these positive findings, this study was extended with a 4-year follow-up[74] to establish the long-term effects of GH therapy in HF. At 48 months, GH replacement therapy was still associated with a significant reductions of LV end-diastolic and end-systolic volumes, and circumferential wall stress, with LV reverse remodeling accordingly, resulting in an increase in LVEF. Further, in the GH group, the improvement of peak Vo_2 was remarkable (final treatment effect of 7.1 ± 0.7 mL/kg/min in the GH group compared with of −1.8 ± 0.5, $P<.001$ in the control group).

In addition, although the study was not designed for hard clinical endpoints, a significant difference in the composite of death and hospitalization for HF was observed. To date, this is the longest study that investigated the effect of GH in CHF.

Further research is needed to verify the efficacy of GH replacement therapy and our group is beginning a randomized double-blind, placebo-controlled trial of GH replacement therapy in CHF patients with coexisting GHD.

Side Effects

General data derived from clinical studies have showed the safety of GH treatment.[75,76] If used with the correct dosage, GH treatment could be considered without major collateral effects. The initial warning of worsening ventricular arrhythmias, perhaps related to the very high dosage of GH used by Frustaci and colleagues,[53] has not been reported by subsequent studies.

It is well-known that an excess of GH, such as in acromegaly, could lead to an increase in ventricular arrhythmia.[77] When all clinical studies were reviewed by Le Corvoisier and colleagues,[12] there were no differences in the incidence of major adverse effects (death, worsening of HF, increased salt retention, and ventricular arrhythmias) between the treatment and placebo arms. Finally, after 48 months of follow-up, Cittadini and colleagues[74] reported no major adverse events in the subjects treated with GH at long-term. In particular, in the final cohort of 17 subjects, only 2 cases of arthralgia, a well-known transient side effect of GH replacement, were reported. The relatively low prevalence of adverse effects observed in this study is in line with data derived from the largest database on GH treatment available.[78]

TESTOSTERONE TREATMENT IN HEART FAILURE
Testosterone Deficiency

The interaction between hormones and cardiac morphology and function is well-recognized,[4,7,11,79,80] with testosterone showing a key role.

Some investigators suggest the hypothesis of a direct action of testosterone on the androgen receptors (ARs) in myocardial cells.[81] Testosterone and its active counterpart dihydrotestosterone (DHEA) interact with AR expressed externally on the cell surface and internally in the cytosol. Extracellular ARs seem to be more linked to the activation of ion channels and signaling pathways. Intracellular ARs are more involved in the androgen target genes modulation, resulting in a fine regulation of myocardial and vascular cell activity.[82] Additionally, there is evidence that the metabolic profile is affected by polymorphisms of ARs.[83]

In the general population, the decline in androgen levels with aging contributes to sarcopenia, visceral adiposity deposition, and osteopenia. From the forth decade of life, there is a decrease in serum testosterone level of about 3.5 ng/dL per year (the so-called phenomenon of andropause).[84] A similar decline has been described for circulating F-S levels, from the second-third decade of life.[85]

To date, it is important to underline that the criteria for TD are not widely accepted. Previous guidelines recommended to consider a TD when the morning total testosterone level drops below 300 mg/dL in two or more occasions in presence of consistent symptoms and signs.[86] Current guidelines suggest that if the total testosterone has been measured with an assay that has been certified by an accuracy-based standardization or quality control program (eg, Centers for Disease Control and Prevention (CDC)) clinicians can use as the lower reference range for total testosterone in healthy, nonobese young men (aged 19–39 years) a value of 264 using the 2.5th percentile, or 303 using the 5th percentile (with a preference for the first one value).[87] In patients whose serum TT concentrations are just above or below the lower limit of normal (eg, 200–400 ng/dL), clinicians should also measure free testosterone. It is important to underline that low testosterone concentrations without symptoms or signs of TD do not establish a diagnosis of hypogonadism. Diagnosing TD in the elderly is challenging due to the significant overlap of signs and symptoms with those of normal aging. Epidemiologic studies demonstrated that the incidence of hypogonadal levels of testosterone in men is 20% in people 60 or older and 30% in 70 or older.[88] Independent groups have showed that TD in older men is associated with an increased risk of death[89,90] supporting the finding that low serum testosterone levels might be used as a marker of poor survival.[89]

It has been demonstrated that the prevalence of TD in patients with CHF syndrome is about 25% to 30%[17,18,23,91–93] associated with an impairment of skeletal muscle function and cardiovascular performance[94] and contributes to the negative outcome.[95–97] In addition, decreased circulating levels of dehydroisoandrosterone sulphate are able to predict mortality in elderly.[98] Recently, Enina and colleagues[99] demonstrated that testosterone levels could be useful as predictors of cardiac resynchronization therapy response in male HF patients.

TD has also been linked to the dysregulation of other metabolic profiles. The association between testosterone and the lipid profile is still a matter of debate but there is some evidence that testosterone inhibits the evolution of preadipocytes into mature adipocytes, thus reducing total fat mass and increasing net lean mass.[100,101] Current evidences suggest that the effects of testosterone on the regulation and on the expression of lipid metabolism are tissue-specific, with the final result of reduced fat deposition in sites such as the arterial wall and the liver.[102] However, testosterone improves IR; there is evidence that those with low testosterone levels have an increased risk of metabolic syndrome and new onset type 2 diabetes.[103,104]

Testosterone Treatment

Taking into account the relationship between testosterone and the cardiovascular system, several studies have investigated the role of testosterone in the treatment of CHF[105] (**Table 2**).

Pugh and colleagues[106] conducted a study on 12 stable male subjects to assess the effects of testosterone in HF. In particular, using a pulmonary flotation catheter, central hemodynamics were measured over 6 hours after administration of a single dose of testosterone (60 mg orally) on 2 consecutive days. An increase in cardiac output in the active arm was observed. Of note, the effects were more evident in subjects with a lower baseline circulating testosterone level and no side effects were reported.

This research continued a few years later with a double-blind, placebo-controlled trial, enrolling 20 male CHF subjects.[95] In this trial, the treatment group (100 mg every 2 weeks for 12 weeks) displayed a significant improvement in the 6-minute walking test (6MWT), in particular in the maximum distance, and in quality of life, assessed by the Minnesota Living with Heart Failure Questionnaire (MLWHFQ). The same group performed a further larger randomized, double-blind, placebo-controlled study involving 76 CHF subjects.[107] In the active group (5 mg/d administered by an adhesive skin patch), the investigators demonstrated a clinical improvement as testified to by the decrease of at least 1 NYHA class (30% of subjects in treated arm vs 8% in untreated). Even if testosterone did not change LV morphology or function, a significant improvement in cardiovascular performance was demonstrated (ie, shuttle walk distance). With regard to QT duration, despite that in a previous report the same group showed that testosterone therapy was able to reduce QT duration[108] and these data were confirmed by a subsequent study by an independent group,[109] no effects of testosterone on QT duration were observed in this larger cohort.

Reassuringly, no significant effects were observed with regard to skeletal muscle bulk and strength, weight, and other cardiovascular parameters (eg, heart rate and blood pressure). In line with a previous report,[110] in which different methods of testosterone administration were tested (ie, acute vs chronic and either via transdermal patch or intramuscular injection), no differences were detected with regard to circulating concentrations of cytokines (eg, tumor necrosis factor [TNF]-α, interleukin [IL]-1β, and IL-6).[70]

To further explore this, Mirdamadi and colleagues[111] performed a double-blind, placebo-controlled trial, involving 50 male subjects. The treatment group received an intramuscular long-acting androgen injection (1 mL of testosterone enanthate 250 mg/mL) once every 4 weeks for 1 to 5 months. They displayed a significantly increased trend in the 6MWT distance and in quality of life scores.

However, recently Navarro-Penalver and colleagues[112] performed a prospective, randomized, double-blind, placebo-controlled, and parallel-group trial comparing testosterone with placebo in males with HFrEF and TD on 25 CHF subjects. Their findings were not consistent with previous reports. Indeed, after 12 months of long-acting intramuscular testosterone administration, clinical symptoms (eg, NYHA class, MLWHFQ score), functional capacity (eg, 6MWT, LVEF), nor other secondary parameters (NT-proBNP levels, lipid profile, body mass index) were observed to improve. With regard to safety, the prostate-specific antigen (PSA) levels did not change and no other adverse side effects were observed.

In the elderly, paraphysiological decrease of skeletal muscle strength, resulting in early fatigue and reduced exercise tolerance, is well-known.[113,114] With this in mind, Caminiti and colleagues[115] performed a double-blind, randomized, placebo-controlled study focused on elderly subjects with stable CHF (median age 70 years). In this trial, the investigators demonstrated that testosterone treatment (12 weeks with very-long-acting intramuscular 1000 mg testosterone undecanoate) improved functional exercise capacity and muscle strength. Of note, peak Vo_2 and index of muscular strength (eg, peak torque and quadriceps maximal intentional contraction) improved in the active group, whereas no effects were observed in the placebo group. Glucose tolerance (expressed as homeostatic model assessment-IR) and baroreflex sensitivity also showed a significant improvement.

The role of exercise rehabilitation in HF is recognized worldwide.[116] Stout and colleagues[117] investigated the effect of testosterone

Table 2
Summary of studies on testosterone treatment in heart failure

First Author, Year	Sample Size (Number)	Gender (%)	Mean Age (Years)	Baseline NYHA Class (Mean ± Sd)	TD	Testosterone Supplementation	Type of Trial	Trial Duration
Pugh et al,[106] 2003	12	Male	NR	NR	NR	60 mg orally day 1 and day 2	R, DB, PC	2 d
Malkin et al,[108] 2003	20	Male	61.5	2.5 ± 0.5	NR	Sustanon 100 mg IM every 2 wk	R, DB, PC	12 wk
Pugh et al,[95] 2004	20	Male	62	NR	NR	Sustanon 100 mg IM every 2 wk	R, DB, PC	12 wk
Malkin et al,[107] 2006	76	Male	64	2.46 ± 0.6	NR	Androderm 5 mg every 24 h	R, DB, PC	12 mo
Caminiti et al,[115] 2009	70	Male	70	2.46 ± 0.5	NR	Long-acting testosterone undecanoate (Nebido) IM at 0, 6, 12 wk	R, DB, PC	12 wk
Iellamo et al,[94] 2010	32	Female	68.7	3 ± 0	NR	Transdermal testosterone	R, DB, PC	6 mo
Schwartz et al,[109] 2011	84	Male (69%) and Female (31%)	70.35	NR	NR	Male: long-acting testosterone undecanoate 1000 mg IM at 0, 6, 12 wk Female: transdermal testosterone 33 mcg (Intrinsa)	R, DB, PC	12 wk

(continued on next page)

Table 2
(continued)

First Author, Year	Sample Size (Number)	Gender (%)	Mean Age (Years)	Baseline NYHA Class (Mean ± Sd)	TD	Testosterone Supplementation	Type of Trial	Trial Duration
Stout et al,[117] 2012	41	Male	67.2	2.5 ± 0.5	low testosterone status	Sustanon 100 mg IM every 2 wk	R, DB, PC	12 wk
Mirdamadi et al,[111] 2014	50	Male	60	2.38 ± 0.57	NR	Long-acting testosterone enanthate 250 mg IM every 4 wk	R, DB, PC	12 wk
Dos Santos et al,[118] 2016	39	Male	51	3	TD	Long-acting testosterone undecylate IM	R	48 wk
Navarro-Penalver et al,[112] 2018	29	Male	64.5	2.3 ± 0.47	TD	Long-acting undecanoate testosterone 1000 mg, IM at 0 and then every 3 mo	R, DB, PC	12 mo

Abbreviations: DB, double blind; IM, intramuscular; NR, not reported; PC, placebo-controlled; R, randomized; sc, subcutaneous; sd, standard deviation.

supplementation when added to a program of exercise rehabilitation. In this report, 28 male subjects with CHF and low testosterone status (defined as <432 ng/dL), were randomly allocated to exercise with testosterone or exercise with placebo. Testosterone treatment (an intramuscular (gluteal) injection of 100 mg testosterone/mL once a fortnight for 12 weeks) induced positive changes of TD symptoms, with improvements in aerobic fitness, leg strength, and depression. These effects were not observed in the placebo group. Following this, an interesting study by Dos Santos and colleagues[118] investigating male subjects with advanced CHF (NYHA class III) and TD were randomized to 3 arms: cycloergometer training, testosterone (intramuscular injection of testosterone undecylate), or both. The investigators not only confirmed beneficial effects of testosterone when added to an exercise training in subjects with CHF but also supported the concept that the peripheral action of testosterone is the main reason for the improvement in cardiovascular performance, providing novel information about the effects of the combined therapies on total body composition, cardiovascular performance, hormonal status, and quality of life.

Current cardiovascular research asks how and whether sex and gender differences are able to modify outcomes.[5,41,119–122] The effect of testosterone treatment was investigated in 36 female subjects treated with testosterone (300 mg, patch transdermal, twice per week). In this study, an improvement in 6MWT distance and in peak V_{O_2} consumption were observed, with a positive effect on metabolic parameters (eg, IR).[94] A separate study of female subjects demonstrated a direct effect of testosterone in the ventricular repolarization in vivo (a shortening effect).[109]

Meta-analysis performed by Toma and colleagues[14] demonstrated that testosterone supplementation in subjects with CHF is associated with a clinically significant improvement in cardiovascular performance, expressed as 6MWT distance, V_{O_2} peak, and NYHA class. Of note, this improvement was superior when compared with the effect of other CHF treatment strategies (eg, beta blockers and angiotensin-converting-enzyme inhibitors).

A few years later, Wang and colleagues[15] performed a meta-analysis that included 8 trials. The investigators showed that testosterone treatment significantly improved exercise capacity (6MWT and shuttle distance), muscle strength, and electrocardiogram indicators (ie, decreased QT intervals) but did not significantly change EF, NT-proBNP, clinical parameters (ie, blood pressure and heart rate), and inflammatory markers (ie, TNF-α, high-sensitivity C-reactive protein, and IL-6).

Side Effects

None of the trials for testosterone replacement showed safety concerns. No major events were reported associated with the treatment[14,15] and there were no significant changes in PSA assays. Skin reactions were described in the studies using topical testosterone but were transient and not severe. Testosterone treatment could be considered safe in HF.

CLINICAL PERSPECTIVES

A growing body of evidence led to the hypothesis that CHF could be considered as a multiple hormone deficiency syndrome. It has been demonstrated that deficiencies in the main anabolic axes cannot be considered as mere epiphenomena and are very common in HF, with a clear association with poor cardiovascular performance and outcomes. Among these, GHD and TD play a pivotal role, and the replacement treatment is an innovative therapy that should be considered in CHF. A prospective multicenter clinical registry, the Trattamento Ormonale nello Scompenso CArdiaco (TOSCA), will investigate this issue.[7,123]

Several points need further discussion. First, it is important to underline that, to date, different patient populations and different routes and dosage of hormone replacement treatment have been tested. Second, all studies only involved subjects with reduced EF and no data are available regarding patients with mildly reduced or preserved EF. Third, due to the short-term nature of most trials, there is a paucity of data regarding strong endpoints (eg, mortality and/or hospitalization).

With regard to GHD, the latest American Heart Association statement on management of dilated cardiomyopathies[124] recommends, with a strong level of consensus, that GHD should be investigated in patients with dilated cardiomyopathy when other signs and/or symptoms of this clinical disorders are present (level of evidence C). They recommend that treatment of the primary disorder be given to all patients with coexisting DCM.

Another consideration is that basal testosterone status (ie, TD) was used in only a few studies as a parameter of enrollment. Recently, in the context of HD in CHF,[41,65,123,125,126] the idea that hormone treatment should be used only when a deficit of the axis of interest is diagnosed rather than in all patients, represents a paradigm shift and has improved the overall outcome. To date, this represents the most promising question in this field.[9,10,19,74] With this in mind, a flowchart to manage the GHD in

Treatment	Target organ	Main effects

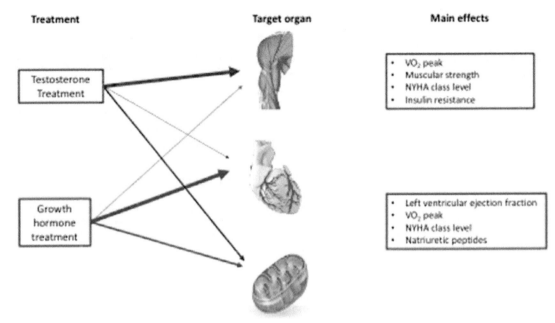

Fig. 1. Effects of testosterone treatment (*blue arrows*) and growth hormone treatment (*orange arrows*). The weight of the arrows indicates the impact of the treatment with regard to the target organ: muscle, heart, and metabolism.

CHF patients has been developed and suggested for clinical use.[76]

SUMMARY

The use of GH and testosterone in the treatment of CHF is promising and in need of further review. Considering all the literature and the authors' own experiences, some suggestions can be considered:

1. GH status and testosterone status should be investigated in all CHF patients, in particular in those who displays signs and/or symptoms of these conditions.
2. GH and testosterone should be administered only in those patients with an impairment of GH or IGF-1 status (eg, GHD) or androgens (ie, TD) as a replacement therapy.
3. An individualized dose titration of GH and testosterone should be considered for each patient depending on clinical and neurohormonal response.

Considering this high frequency of multiple HD in CHF, no data are available regarding combined hormone treatment. This is important, considering that these 2 treatments seem to exert different action on cardiovascular system: GH being more effective on the central pathophysiological mechanisms and testosterone more effective on the peripheral mechanisms (**Fig. 1**).

REFERENCES

1. Ponikowski P, Voors AA, Anker SD, et al. 2016 ESC guidelines for the diagnosis and treatment of acute and chronic heart failure: the task force for the diagnosis and treatment of acute and chronic heart failure of the European Society of Cardiology (ESC). Developed with the special contribution of the Heart Failure Association (HFA) of the ESC. Eur J Heart Fail 2016;18:891–975.
2. Braunwald E. Heart failure. JACC Heart Fail 2013; 1:1–20.
3. Mann DL, Bristow MR. Mechanisms and models in heart failure: the biomechanical model and beyond. Circulation 2005;111:2837–49.
4. Marra AM, Improda N, Capalbo D, et al. Cardiovascular abnormalities and impaired exercise performance in adolescents with congenital adrenal hyperplasia. J Clin Endocrinol Metab 2015;100: 644–52.
5. Salzano A, Demelo-Rodriguez P, Marra AM, et al. A focused review of gender differences in antithrombotic therapy. Curr Med Chem 2017;24: 2576–88.
6. Pasquali D, Arcopinto M, Renzullo A, et al. Cardiovascular abnormalities in Klinefelter syndrome. Int J Cardiol 2013;168:754–9.
7. Arcopinto M, Salzano A, Ferrara F, et al. The Tosca registry: an ongoing, observational, multicenter registry for chronic heart failure. Transl Med UniSa 2016;14:21–7.

8. Sacca F, Puorro G, Marsili A, et al. Long-term effect of epoetin alfa on clinical and biochemical markers in friedreich ataxia. Mov Disord 2016;31:734–41.

9. Arcopinto M, Salzano A, Isgaard J, et al. Hormone replacement therapy in heart failure. Curr Opin Cardiol 2015;30:277–84.

10. Napoli R, Salzano A, Bossone E, et al. Hormonal therapy in the treatment of chronic heart failure A2 - Vasan, Ramachandran S. In: Sawyer DB, editor. Encyclopedia of cardiovascular research and medicine. Oxford: Elsevier; 2018. p. 508–16.

11. Marra AM, Bobbio E, D'Assante R, et al. Growth hormone as biomarker in heart failure. Heart Fail Clin 2018;14:65–74.

12. Le Corvoisier P, Hittinger L, Chanson P, et al. Cardiac effects of growth hormone treatment in chronic heart failure: a meta-analysis. J Clin Endocrinol Metab 2007;92:180–5.

13. Tritos NA, Danias PG. Growth hormone therapy in congestive heart failure due to left ventricular systolic dysfunction: a meta-analysis. Endocr Pract 2008;14:40–9.

14. Toma M, McAlister FA, Coglianese EE, et al. Testosterone supplementation in heart failure: a meta-analysis. Circ Heart Fail 2012;5:315–21.

15. Wang W, Jiang T, Li C, et al. Will testosterone replacement therapy become a new treatment of chronic heart failure? A review based on 8 clinical trials. J Thorac Dis 2016;8:E269–77.

16. Broglio F, Benso A, Gottero C, et al. Patients with dilated cardiomyopathy show reduction of the somatotroph responsiveness to GHRH both alone and combined with arginine. Eur J Endocrinol 2000;142:157–63.

17. Arcopinto M, Salzano A, Bossone E, et al. Multiple hormone deficiencies in chronic heart failure. Int J Cardiol 2015;184:421–3.

18. Salzano A, Marra AM, Ferrara F, et al. Multiple hormone deficiency syndrome in heart failure with preserved ejection fraction. Int J Cardiol 2016;225: 1–3.

19. Cittadini A, Saldamarco L, Marra AM, et al. Growth hormone deficiency in patients with chronic heart failure and beneficial effects of its correction. J Clin Endocrinol Metab 2009;94:3329–36.

20. Jankowska EA, Biel B, Majda J, et al. Anabolic deficiency in men with chronic heart failure: prevalence and detrimental impact on survival. Circulation 2006;114:1829–37.

21. Niebauer J, Pflaum CD, Clark AL, et al. Deficient insulin-like growth factor I in chronic heart failure predicts altered body composition, anabolic deficiency, cytokine and neurohormonal activation. J Am Coll Cardiol 1998;32:393–7.

22. Arcopinto M, Salzano A, Giallauria F, et al. Growth hormone deficiency is associated with worse cardiac function, physical performance, and outcome

in chronic heart failure: insights from the T.O.S.C.A. GHD study. PLoS One 2017;12:e0170058.

23. Kontoleon PE, Anastasiou-Nana MI, Papapetrou PD, et al. Hormonal profile in patients with congestive heart failure. Int J Cardiol 2003;87:179–83.

24. Petretta M, Colao A, Sardu C, et al. NT-proBNP, IGF-I and survival in patients with chronic heart failure. Growth Horm IGF Res 2007;17:288–96.

25. Anwar A, Gaspoz JM, Pampallona S, et al. Effect of congestive heart failure on the insulin-like growth factor-1 system. Am J Cardiol 2002;90:1402–5.

26. Bolger A, Doehner W, Anker SD. Insulin-like growth factor-I can be helpful towards end of life. BMJ 2001;322:674–5.

27. Anker SD, Volterrani M, Pflaum CD, et al. Acquired growth hormone resistance in patients with chronic heart failure: implications for therapy with growth hormone. J Am Coll Cardiol 2001;38:443–52.

28. Molitch ME, Clemmons DR, Malozowski S, et al. Evaluation and treatment of adult growth hormone deficiency: an Endocrine Society clinical practice guideline. J Clin Endocrinol Metab 2011;96: 1587–609.

29. Ghigo E, Aimaretti G, Corneli G. Diagnosis of adult GH deficiency. Growth Horm IGF Res 2008;18: 1–16.

30. Yuen KC, Tritos NA, Samson SL, et al. American Association of Clinical Endocrinologists and American College of Endocrinology disease state clinical review: update on growth hormone stimulation testing and proposed revised cut-point for the glucagon stimulation test in the diagnosis of adult growth hormone deficiency. Endocr Pract 2016;22:1235–44.

31. Gordon MB, Levy RA, Gut R, et al. Trends in growth hormone stimulation testing and growth hormone dosing in adult growth hormone deficiency patients: results from the answer program. Endocr Pract 2016;22:396–405.

32. Prodam F, Pagano L, Corneli G, et al. Update on epidemiology, etiology, and diagnosis of adult growth hormone deficiency. J Endocrinol Invest 2008;31:6–11.

33. Pena-Bello L, Seoane-Pillado T, Sangiao-Alvarellos S, et al. Oral glucose-stimulated growth hormone (GH) test in adult GH deficiency patients and controls: Potential utility of a novel test. Eur J Intern Med 2017;44:55–61.

34. Rahim A, Toogood AA, Shalet SM. The assessment of growth hormone status in normal young adult males using a variety of provocative agents. Clin Endocrinol (Oxf) 1996;45:557–62.

35. Junnila RK, Strasburger CJ, Bidlingmaier M. Pitfalls of insulin-like growth factor-i and growth hormone assays. Endocrinol Metab Clin North Am 2015;44: 27–34.

36. Colao A, Di Somma C, Cuocolo A, et al. The severity of growth hormone deficiency correlates

with the severity of cardiac impairment in 100 adult patients with hypopituitarism: an observational, case-control study. J Clin Endocrinol Metab 2004; 89:5998–6004.

37. Rosen T, Bengtsson BA. Premature mortality due to cardiovascular disease in hypopituitarism. Lancet 1990;336:285–8.

38. Bhandari SS, Narayan H, Jones DJ, et al. Plasma growth hormone is a strong predictor of risk at 1 year in acute heart failure. Eur J Heart Fail 2016; 18:281–9.

39. Fonarow GC, Adams KF Jr, Abraham WT, et al, ADHERE Scientific Advisory Committee, Study Group, and Investigators. Risk stratification for in-hospital mortality in acutely decompensated heart failure: classification and regression tree analysis. JAMA 2005;293:572–80.

40. Wang CY, Chung HW, Cho NY, et al. Idiopathic growth hormone deficiency in the morphologically normal pituitary gland is associated with perfusion delay. Radiology 2011;258:213–21.

41. Marra AM, Benjamin N, Eichstaedt C, et al. Gender-related differences in pulmonary arterial hypertension targeted drugs administration. Pharmacol Res 2016;114:103–9.

42. Yoshida T, Tabony AM, Galvez S, et al. Molecular mechanisms and signaling pathways of angio-tensin II-induced muscle wasting: potential therapeutic targets for cardiac cachexia. Int J Biochem Cell Biol 2013;45:2322–32.

43. Giustina A, Veldhuis JD. Pathophysiology of the neuroregulation of growth hormone secretion in experimental animals and the human. Endocr Rev 1998;19:717–97.

44. Fazio S, Palmieri EA, Biondi B, et al. The role of the GH-IGF-I axis in the regulation of myocardial growth: from experimental models to human evidence. Eur J Endocrinol 2000;142:211–6.

45. Piccioli L, Arcopinto M, Salzano A, et al. The impairment of the growth hormone/insulin-like growth factor 1 (IGF-1) axis in heart failure: a possible target for future therapy. Monaldi Arch Chest Dis 2018; 88:975.

46. Yang R, Bunting S, Gillett N, et al. Growth hormone improves cardiac performance in experimental heart failure. Circulation 1995;92:262–7.

47. Duerr RL, McKirnan MD, Gim RD, et al. Cardiovascular effects of insulin-like growth factor-1 and growth hormone in chronic left ventricular failure in the rat. Circulation 1996;93:2188–96.

48. Ryoke T, Gu Y, Mao L, et al. Progressive cardiac dysfunction and fibrosis in the cardiomyopathic hamster and effects of growth hormone and angiotensin-converting enzyme inhibition. Circulation 1999;100:1734–43.

49. Cittadini A, Ishiguro Y, Stromer H, et al. Insulin-like growth factor-1 but not growth hormone augments

mammalian myocardial contractility by sensitizing the myofilament to Ca2+ through a wortmannin-sensitive pathway: studies in rat and ferret isolated muscles. Circ Res 1998;83:50–9.

50. Cittadini A, Isgaard J, Monti MG, et al. Growth hormone prolongs survival in experimental postinfarction heart failure. J Am Coll Cardiol 2003;41: 2154–63.

51. Cittadini A, Grossman JD, Napoli R, et al. Growth hormone attenuates early left ventricular remodel-ing and improves cardiac function in rats with large myocardial infarction. J Am Coll Cardiol 1997;29: 1109–16.

52. Fazio S, Sabatini D, Capaldo B, et al. A preliminary study of growth hormone in the treatment of dilated cardiomyopathy. N Engl J Med 1996;334:809–14.

53. Frustaci A, Gentiloni N, Russo MA. Growth hormone in the treatment of dilated cardiomyopathy. N Engl J Med 1996;335:672–3 [author reply: 3–4].

54. Isgaard J, Bergh CH, Caidahl K, et al. A placebo-controlled study of growth hormone in patients with congestive heart failure. Eur Heart J 1998;19: 1704–11.

55. Osterziel KJ, Strohm O, Schuler J, et al. Randomised, double-blind, placebo-controlled trial of human recombinant growth hormone in patients with chronic heart failure due to dilated cardiomyopathy. Lancet 1998;351:1233–7.

56. Genth-Zotz S, Zotz R, Geil S, et al. Recombinant growth hormone therapy in patients with ischemic cardiomyopathy : effects on hemodynamics, left ventricular function, and cardiopulmonary exercise capacity. Circulation 1999;99:18–21.

57. Spallarossa P, Rossettin P, Minuto F, et al. Evaluation of growth hormone administration in patients with chronic heart failure secondary to coronary artery disease. Am J Cardiol 1999;84:430–3.

58. Jose VJ, Zechariah TU, George P, et al. Growth hormone therapy in patients with dilated cardiomyopathy: preliminary observations of a pilot study. Indian Heart J 1999;51:183–5.

59. Smit JW, Janssen YJ, Lamb HJ, et al. Six months of recombinant human GH therapy in patients with ischemic cardiac failure does not influence left ventricular function and mass. J Clin Endocrinol Metab 2001;86:4638–43.

60. Perrot A, Ranke MB, Dietz R, et al. Growth hormone treatment in dilated cardiomyopathy. J Card Surg 2001;16:127–31.

61. Napoli R, Guardasole V, Matarazzo M, et al. Growth hormone corrects vascular dysfunction in patients with chronic heart failure. J Am Coll Cardiol 2002; 39:90–5.

62. Adamopoulos S, Parissis JT, Paraskevaidis I, et al. Effects of growth hormone on circulating cytokine network, and left ventricular contractile performance and geometry in patients with idiopathic

dilated cardiomyopathy. Eur Heart J 2003;24: 2186–96.

63. Acevedo M, Corbalan R, Chamorro G, et al. Administration of growth hormone to patients with advanced cardiac heart failure: effects upon left ventricular function, exercise capacity, and neurohormonal status. Int J Cardiol 2003;87: 185–91.

64. van Thiel SW, Smit JW, de Roos A, et al. Six-months of recombinant human GH therapy in patients with ischemic cardiac failure. Int J Cardiovasc Imaging 2004;20:53–60.

65. Fazio S, Palmieri EA, Affuso F, et al. Effects of growth hormone on exercise capacity and cardio-pulmonary performance in patients with chronic heart failure. J Clin Endocrinol Metab 2007;92: 4218–23.

66. Marra AM, Arcopinto M, Bobbio E, et al. An unusual case of dilated cardiomyopathy associated with partial hypopituitarism. Intern Emerg Med 2012; 7(Suppl 2):S85–7.

67. Frustaci A, Gentiloni N, Corsello SM, et al. Reversible dilated cardiomyopathy due to growth hormone deficiency. Chest 1992;102:326–7.

68. Cuneo R, Salomon F, Wilmshurst P, et al. Reversible dilated cardiomyopathy due to growth hormone deficiency. Am J Clin Pathol 1993;100:585–6.

69. Cittadini A, Ines Comi L, Longobardi S, et al. A preliminary randomized study of growth hormone administration in Becker and Duchenne muscular dystrophies. Eur Heart J 2003;24:664–72.

70. Marra AM, Arcopinto M, Salzano A, et al. Detectable interleukin-9 plasma levels are associated with impaired cardiopulmonary functional capacity and all-cause mortality in patients with chronic heart failure. Int J Cardiol 2016;209:114–7.

71. Brankovic M, Akkerhuis KM, Mouthaan H, et al. Cardiometabolic biomarkers and their temporal patterns predict poor outcome in chronic heart failure (Bio-SHiFT study). J Clin Endocrinol Metab 2018;103:3954–64.

72. Salzano A, Marra AM, Bossone E, et al. Letter to the Editor: "Cardiometabolic biomarkers and their temporal patterns predict poor outcome in chronic heart failure (Bio-SHiFT study)". J Clin Endocrinol Metab 2018;104(3):734–5.

73. Brankovic M, Akkerhuis KM, Umans V, et al. Response to Letter: Cardiometabolic biomarkers and their temporal patterns predict poor outcome in chronic heart failure (Bio-SHiFT study). J Clin Endocrinol Metab 2019;104(3):736–7.

74. Cittadini A, Marra AM, Arcopinto M, et al. Growth hormone replacement delays the progression of chronic heart failure combined with growth hormone deficiency: an extension of a randomized controlled single-blind study. JACC Heart Fail 2013;1:325–30.

75. Isgaard J, Arcopinto M, Karason K, et al. GH and the cardiovascular system: an update on a topic at heart. Endocrine 2015;48:25–35.

76. Salzano A, Marra AM, D'Assante R, et al. Growth hormone therapy in heart failure. Heart Fail Clin 2018;14:501–15.

77. Sacca L, Napoli R, Cittadini A. Growth hormone, acromegaly, and heart failure: an intricate triangulation. Clin Endocrinol (Oxf) 2003;59:660–71.

78. Spielhagen C, Schwahn C, Moller K, et al. The benefit of long-term growth hormone (GH) replacement therapy in hypopituitary adults with GH deficiency: results of the German KIMS database. Growth Horm IGF Res 2011;21:1–10.

79. Salzano A, Rocca A, Arcopinto M, et al. Bowel Angiodysplasia and Myocardial Infarction secondary to an ischaemic imbalance: a case report. Open Med (Wars) 2015;10:543–8.

80. Salzano A, Sirico D, Golia L, et al. [The portopulmonary hypertension: an overview from diagnosis to treatment]. Monaldi Arch Chest Dis 2013;80:66–8.

81. Marsh JD, Lehmann MH, Ritchie RH, et al. Androgen receptors mediate hypertrophy in cardiac myocytes. Circulation 1998;98:256–61.

82. Perusquia M, Stallone JN. Do androgens play a beneficial role in the regulation of vascular tone? Nongenomic vascular effects of testosterone metabolites. Am J Physiol Heart Circ Physiol 2010; 298:H1301–7.

83. Tirabassi G, Cutini M, Beltrami B, et al. Androgen receptor GGC repeat might be more involved than CAG repeat in the regulation of the metabolic profile in men. Intern Emerg Med 2016;11:1067–75.

84. Lapauw B, Goemaere S, Zmierczak H, et al. The decline of serum testosterone levels in community-dwelling men over 70 years of age: descriptive data and predictors of longitudinal changes. Eur J Endocrinol 2008;159:459–68.

85. Kaufman JM, Vermeulen A. The decline of androgen levels in elderly men and its clinical and therapeutic implications. Endocr Rev 2005; 26:833–76.

86. Bhasin S, Cunningham GR, Hayes FJ, et al. Testosterone therapy in men with androgen deficiency syndromes: an Endocrine Society clinical practice guideline. J Clin Endocrinol Metab 2010;95: 2536–59.

87. Bhasin S, Brito JP, Cunningham GR, et al. Testosterone therapy in men with hypogonadism: an endocrine society clinical practice guideline. J Clin Endocrinol Metab 2018;103:1715–44.

88. Harman SM, Metter EJ, Tobin JD, et al, Baltimore Longitudinal Study of Aging. Longitudinal effects of aging on serum total and free testosterone levels in healthy men. Baltimore Longitudinal Study of Aging. J Clin Endocrinol Metab 2001;86: 724–31.

89. Haring R, Volzke H, Steveling A, et al. Low serum testosterone levels are associated with increased risk of mortality in a population-based cohort of men aged 20-79. Eur Heart J 2010;31:1494–501.

90. Laughlin GA, Barrett-Connor E, Bergstrom J. Low serum testosterone and mortality in older men. J Clin Endocrinol Metab 2008;93:68–75.

91. Anker SD, Chua TP, Ponikowski P, et al. Hormonal changes and catabolic/anabolic imbalance in chronic heart failure and their importance for cardiac cachexia. Circulation 1997;96:526–34.

92. Moriyama Y, Yasue H, Yoshimura M, et al. The plasma levels of dehydroepiandrosterone sulfate are decreased in patients with chronic heart failure in proportion to the severity. J Clin Endocrinol Metab 2000;85:1834–40.

93. Malkin CJ, Jones TH, Channer KS. Testosterone in chronic heart failure. Front Horm Res 2009;37:183–96.

94. Iellamo F, Volterrani M, Caminiti G, et al. Testosterone therapy in women with chronic heart failure: a pilot double-blind, randomized, placebo-controlled study. J Am Coll Cardiol 2010;56:1310–6.

95. Pugh PJ, Jones RD, West JN, et al. Testosterone treatment for men with chronic heart failure. Heart 2004;90:446–7.

96. Malkin CJ, Channer KS, Jones TH. Testosterone and heart failure. Curr Opin Endocrinol Diabetes Obes 2010;17:262–8.

97. Volterrani M, Rosano G, Iellamo F. Testosterone and heart failure. Endocrine 2012;42:272–7.

98. Ohlsson C, Labrie F, Barrett-Connor E, et al. Low serum levels of dehydroepiandrosterone sulfate predict all-cause and cardiovascular mortality in elderly Swedish men. J Clin Endocrinol Metab 2010;95:4406–14.

99. Enina T, Kuznetsov V, Soldatova A, et al. Association of sex hormones level and effect of cardiac resynchronisation therapy in men with congestive heart failure. Dis Markers 2018;2018.

100. Gupta V, Bhasin S, Guo W, et al. Effects of dihydrotestosterone on differentiation and proliferation of human mesenchymal stem cells and preadipocytes. Mol Cell Endocrinol 2008;296:32–40.

101. Filippi S, Vignozzi L, Morelli A, et al. Testosterone partially ameliorates metabolic profile and erectile responsiveness to PDE5 inhibitors in an animal model of male metabolic syndrome. J Sex Med 2009;6:3274–88.

102. Kelly DM, Akhtar S, Sellers DJ, et al. Testosterone differentially regulates targets of lipid and glucose metabolism in liver, muscle and adipose tissues of the testicular feminised mouse. Endocrine 2016;54:504–15.

103. Oh JY, Barrett-Connor E, Wedick NM, et al. Endogenous sex hormones and the development of type 2 diabetes in older men and women: the Rancho Bernardo study. Diabetes Care 2002;25:55–60.

104. Brand JS, Rovers MM, Yeap BB, et al. Testosterone, sex hormone-binding globulin and the metabolic syndrome in men: an individual participant data meta-analysis of observational studies. PLoS One 2014;9:e100409.

105. D'Assante R, Piccioli L, Valente P, et al. Testosterone treatment in chronic heart failure. Review of literature and future perspectives. Monaldi Arch Chest Dis 2018;88:976.

106. Pugh PJ, Jones TH, Channer KS. Acute haemodynamic effects of testosterone in men with chronic heart failure. Eur Heart J 2003;24:909–15.

107. Malkin CJ, Pugh PJ, West JN, et al. Testosterone therapy in men with moderate severity heart failure: a double-blind randomized placebo controlled trial. Eur Heart J 2006;27:57–64.

108. Malkin CJ, Morris PD, Pugh PJ, et al. Effect of testosterone therapy on QT dispersion in men with heart failure. Am J Cardiol 2003;92:1241–3.

109. Schwartz JB, Volterrani M, Caminiti G, et al. Effects of testosterone on the Q-T interval in older men and older women with chronic heart failure. Int J Androl 2011;34:e415–21.

110. Pugh PJ, Jones RD, Malkin CJ, et al. Physiologic testosterone therapy has no effect on serum levels of tumour necrosis factor-alpha in men with chronic heart failure. Endocr Res 2005;31:271–83.

111. Mirdamadi A, Garakyaraghi M, Pourmoghaddas A, et al. Beneficial effects of testosterone therapy on functional capacity, cardiovascular parameters, and quality of life in patients with congestive heart failure. Biomed Res Int 2014;2014:392432.

112. Navarro-Penalver M, Perez-Martinez MT, Gomez-Bueno M, et al. Testosterone replacement therapy in deficient patients with chronic heart failure: a randomized double-blind controlled pilot study. J Cardiovasc Pharmacol Ther 2018;23:543–50.

113. Dharmarajan K, Rich MW. Epidemiology, pathophysiology, and prognosis of heart failure in older adults. Heart Fail Clin 2017;13:417–26.

114. Panjrath G, Ahmed A. Diagnosis and management of heart failure in older adults. Heart Fail Clin 2017;13:427–44.

115. Caminiti G, Volterrani M, Iellamo F, et al. Effect of long-acting testosterone treatment on functional exercise capacity, skeletal muscle performance, insulin resistance, and baroreflex sensitivity in elderly patients with chronic heart failure a double-blind, placebo-controlled, randomized study. J Am Coll Cardiol 2009;54:919–27.

116. Pedretti RFE, Fattirolli F, Griffo R, et al. Cardiac Prevention and Rehabilitation "3.0": from acute to chronic phase. Position Paper of the Italian

Association for Cardiovascular Prevention and Rehabilitation (GICR-IACPR). Monaldi Arch Chest Dis 2018;88:1004.

117. Stout M, Tew GA, Doll H, et al. Testosterone therapy during exercise rehabilitation in male patients with chronic heart failure who have low testosterone status: a double-blind randomized controlled feasibility study. Am Heart J 2012;164: 893–901.

118. Dos Santos MR, Sayegh AL, Bacurau AV, et al. Effect of exercise training and testosterone replacement on skeletal muscle wasting in patients with heart failure with testosterone deficiency. Mayo Clin Proc 2016;91:575–86.

119. Marra AM, Biskup E, Raparelli V, et al. The Internal Medicine and Assessment of Gender Differences in Europe (IMAGINE): The new European Federation of Internal Medicine initiative on sex and gender medicine. Eur J Intern Med 2018;51: e30–2.

120. Salzano A, Proietti M, D'Assante R, et al. Bleeding related to non-vitamin K antagonist oral anticoagulants in emergency department: A "Real-world" snapshot from Southern Italy. On behalf of MIRC-NOAC study group. Eur J Intern Med 2018;48: e21–4.

121. Bossone E, Lyon A, Citro R, et al. Takotsubo cardiomyopathy: an integrated multi-imaging approach. Eur Heart J Cardiovasc Imaging 2014;15:366–77.

122. Marra AM, Salzano A, Arcopinto M, et al. The impact of gender in cardiovascular medicine: Lessons from the gender/sex-issue in heart failure. Monaldi Arch Chest Dis 2018;88:988.

123. Bossone E, Arcopinto M, Iacoviello M, et al, TOSCA Investigators. Multiple hormonal and metabolic deficiency syndrome in chronic heart failure: rationale, design, and demographic characteristics of the T.O.S.CA. Registry. Intern Emerg Med 2018; 13(5):661–71.

124. Bozkurt B, Colvin M, Cook J, et al. Current diagnostic and treatment strategies for specific dilated cardiomyopathies: a scientific statement from the American Heart Association. Circulation 2016; 134:e579–646.

125. Bossone E, Limongelli G, Malizia G, et al. The T.O.S.CA. project: research, education and care. Monaldi Arch Chest Dis 2011;76:198–203.

126. Cittadini A, Monti MG, Castiello MC, et al. Insulin-like growth factor-1 protects from vascular stenosis and accelerates re-endothelialization in a rat model of carotid artery injury. J Thromb Haemost 2009;7: 1920–8.

The Management of Thyroid Abnormalities in Chronic Heart Failure

Bernadette Biondi, MD

KEYWORDS

- Hypothyroidism • Low T3 syndrome • Heart failure • Cardiac fetal phenotype • Levothyroxine
- liothyronine

KEY POINTS

- Normal triiodothyronine (T3) levels are essential to preserve cardiac morphology and function.
- Overt and subclinical hypothyroidism are associated with an increased risk of heart failure, and levothyroxine is able to improve cardiovascular function in hypothyroid patients.
- Low T3 syndrome can develop in patients with advanced heart failure and is associated with a negative prognosis.
- Low T3 syndrome is associated with alterations in thyroid hormone receptors expression, contributing to the development of a cardiac fetal phenotype, leading to cardiac dysfunction.
- The positive effects of treatment with thyroid hormones in patients with low T3 and heart failure support their potential therapeutic approach in heart failure.

INTRODUCTION

It is widely recognized that thyroid hormone (TH) excess (overt hyperthyroidism and subclinical hyperthyroidism) and TH deficiency (overt hypothyroidism and subclinical hypothyroidism [SHypo]) can represent potential causes of the onset or worsening of heart failure (HF).[1–3] Moreover, changes in thyroid function can develop in acute and chronic illnesses (nonthyroidal illnesses), including HF.[4,5]

CELLULAR MECHANISMS OF THYROID HORMONE ACTION ON THE HEART

Triiodothyronine (T3), the active TH, affects heart rate, cardiac contractility, and systemic vascular resistance (SVR).[1,4,5] The physiologic effects of T3 on the cardiovascular (CV) system are in part mediated by genomic mechanisms, which result from the binding of T3 to nuclear TH receptors (TRs).[4,6] These receptors, which are abundant in the human atria and ventricles, regulate the transcription of various cardiac genes expression, ion channels, and cell surface receptors. The transcriptions of α–myosin heavy chain (MHC) isoform, sarcoplasmic reticulum Ca^{2+}-adenosine triphosphatase ATPase (SERCA2), voltage-gated K^+ channels, β_1-adrenergic receptors, guanine nucleotide regulatory proteins, adenylate cyclase, NA^+/K^+-ATPase, atrial brain natriuretic peptide (BNP), and malic enzyme are up-regulated by T3.[1,4,5] On the contrary, the expressions of β-MHC, phospholamban, Na^+/Ca^{2+} exchanger, TR-α1, and adenylyl cyclase types V and VI are down-regulated by T3.[1,4,5] Nongenomic TH actions, which do not involve TR-mediated transcriptional events, are more rapid than genomic effects; they control the effects of T3 on the transport of glucose and amino acids and ion fluxes across the plasma

Disclosure Statement: The author has nothing to disclose.
Department of Clinical Medicine and Surgery, University of Naples Federico II, Via Sergio Pansini 5, Naples 80131, Italy
E-mail addresses: bebiondi@unina.it; bebiondi@libero.it

Heart Failure Clin 15 (2019) 393–398
https://doi.org/10.1016/j.hfc.2019.02.008
1551-7136/19/© 2019 Elsevier Inc. All rights reserved.

membrane; they also regulate the cytoskeleton and mitochondrial functions.[4,6]

Altogether, these direct and indirect effects of TH are important in regulating the cardiac rhythm and CV hemodynamic. Genomic and nongenomic TH actions control the cardiac pacemaker and heart rate, the potential duration and repolarization currents, the response to β-adrenergic receptor, and the interaction with other neurohormonal factors.[1,4,7] Moreover, T3 administration is able to improve the CV hemodynamic by influencing the relaxation and contractile properties of the myocardium and by acting on the cardiac preload and afterload.[1,7] Cardiac volume is increased by T3 administration for the activation of the renin-angiotensin-aldosterone system (RASS); on the contrary, cardiac afterload is reduced because of the T3 effects on the vascular tone.[4] T3 reduces SVR and increases nitric oxide availability, improving endothelial function.[4,5]

THYROID DYSFUNCTION AND HEART FAILURE

Overt hypothyroidism (characterized by increased serum thyrotropin [TSH] and reduced free T3 and free thyroxine levels) is associated with left ventricular diastolic dysfunction.[8] The activity of the Ca^{2+}-ATPase within the sarcoplasmic reticulum is decreased, with a consequent reduced reuptake of calcium during diastole.[7,8] Moreover, both systolic and diastolic functions are impaired during effort, leading to an decreased exercise tolerance for the slowed myocardial relaxation and the impaired left ventricular filling and vasodilatation during effort.[9,10] The onset of dyspnea during exercise can be the first symptom of the altered CV hemodynamic in patients with TH deficiency.[9,10]

CV findings, similar to overt hypothyroidism, also have been reported in patients with SHypo, a condition characterized by increased serum TSH with levels of THs within the reference range, although at their lower limits.[2,3] Several studies using Doppler echocardiography, tissue Doppler, and cardiac MRI suggest that patients with mild TH deficiency or severe TH deficiency can have CV alterations, leading to a higher risk of developing HF when TH deficiency is untreated in the long-term.[2,3,9–14] Moreover, SHypo can be a risk factor for cardiac death in patients with chronic HF.[15]

Treatment of overt hypothyroidism and SHypo with levothyroxine (LT4) is able to prevent the progressive left ventricle dysfunction and improve systolic and diastolic dysfunctions, SVR, and endothelial function, improve cardiac output thereby increasing (CO) and stroke volume.[11,12,16] Therefore, LT4 in replacement doses is recommended by international guidelines and expert opinions in patients with serum TSH above 10 mU/L.[2,3,17,18] This treatment also should be considered when serum TSH is persistently increased in mild disease (TSH 4.5–9.9 mU/L), especially in patients with a high CV background.[2,3,17,18]

THYROID ABNORMALITIES IN NONTHYROIDAL ILLNESS SYNDROME

Nonthyroidal illness syndrome (NTIS) is characterized by decreased serum T3 levels, normal to high levels of reverse T3 (rT3), and inappropriately normal serum TSH or low serum TSH.[19–21] This syndrome can be considered a neuroendocrine response to a severe illness or starvation. Initial abnormalities of NTIS are characterized by decreased serum T3 and increased rT3 levels.[19,20] The pathophysiologic basis of the development of these alterations are related to the following effects: (1) a decreased extrathyroidal conversion of thyroxin (T4) to T3 for the reduced activity of type 2 deiodinase, (2) a decreased transport of T4, and (3) an increased TH catabolism for the enhanced activity of type 3 deiodinase (D3) in the peripheral tissues.[19–22] rT3 is consequently increased due to its reduced peripheral catabolism and clearance.

TSH levels may rise briefly after the onset of the acute disease; however, circulating TSH levels usually remain within the low to normal range. Subsequently, TSH can be decreased as a consequence of a central hypothyroidism due to a reduced serum TSH secretion for abnormalities in thyrotropin-releasing hormone secretion and clearance. The progressive development of a low serum T4 is linked to an increased probability of death.[19–22]

Low levels of T3 are associated with a decreased metabolic rate. Therefore, the changes in TH homeostasis during the acute phase of NTIS have been interpreted as an attempt to save energy expenditure and do not require any intervention. This interpretation of the low T3 syndrome, however, remains controversial and has been debated for many years probably because it may have a different significance in the acute and chronic phases of illness.[21]

Experts suggest that serum TSH and T3 levels should be reassessed within 1 months to 3 months after an acute illness before deciding to start a treatment with replacement doses of TH.[17,19–22]

THYROID ABNORMALITIES IN HEART FAILURE

HF represents a common final condition of severe cardiac diseases.[23]

At the beginning of its onset, HF is characterized by a decreased CO, increased atrial pressure, and inadequate blood volume, which is compensated by the activation of the RAAS and systemic nervous system to preserve blood volume and pressure. A low T3 syndrome can develop in this phase of HF; it could represent an adaptive process to reduce energy expenditure and metabolic demand. Subsequently, the progression of HF is characterized by a persistent neuroendocrine activation, which is associated with an increase in hormonal response (enhanced levels of RAAS, vasopressin, cortisol, insulin, atrial natriuretic peptide, and BNP and reduced levels of growth hormone) and in inflammatory and immunologic mediators (cytokines, such as interleukin 6 and tumor necrosis factor). All these changes are responsible for an increased cardiac overload and myocardial fibrosis with a negative cardiac remodeling and a progressive deterioration and apoptosis of myocytes and endothelial function. In this advanced stage of HF, the administration of β-adrenergic blocking drugs, digitalis, angiotensin-converting enzyme inhibitors, diuretics, and aldosterone antagonists can improve symptoms and CO. Morbidity, mortality, and recurrent hospitalization, however, are always high in patients with advanced HF for the progressive and irreversible cachexia.[23] Therefore, the persistent activation of the hormonal and inflammatory system and the persistent low T3 syndrome represent a maladaptive mechanism inducing cellular, functional, and morphologic negative CV changes with a negative cardiac remodeling. All these factors are responsible for the progression of HF and death.

In physiologic conditions, TH controls cardiac growth and maturation; its deficiency in the low T3 syndrome is associated with alterations in expression of TRs, contributing to the development of a cardiac fetal phenotype, leading to cardiac dysfunction.[24–29]

The hypoxia and the inflammatory response to HF are able to reduce the type 2 deiodinase activity in the cardiomyocytes, which results in a decrease of intracellular T3 bioavailability.[24] Changes in the deiodinase activities are associated with the increase in proinflammatory cytokines; they can modulate the cardiac levels of T3, contributing to a local low T3 state in the failing heart. Hypoxia also is able to induce the expression of D3 in cardiomyocytes. In a rat model of right ventricular (RV) hypertrophy and failure, D3 activity increased in the chronically overloaded RV, whereas no changes were observed in the LV of the same heart.[25]

The abnormalities in TRs and the decreased deiodinase activities could both lead to the development of important changes in cardiac gene expression, which are similar to those observed in hypothyroidism. The induction of D3 in the cardiomyocytes is associated with a decrease in the T3 concentrations in the tissue and in the T3-dependent gene expression with TRα 1 overexpression.[26–29] In a rat model of starvation-induced low T3 syndrome, the mRNA content of the α-MHC and SERCA2 was reduced.[27,29,30] Propylthiouracil-induced hypothyroidism in rats was responsible for a reduction of the myocyte cross-sectional area, leading to cardiac atrophy. Similarly, T3 deficiency induces alterations in the myocyte shape typical of progressive HF.[31,32] Therefore, long-term T3 deficiency is responsible for the negative effects on myocardial function, histology, and morphology, inducing cellular fibrosis and a negative cardiac remodeling with cellular and structural changes similar to those observed in the progression of HF[31,32] (**Table 1**). All these findings suggest that T3 has an important role in regulating myocyte transverse shape and wall stress and could play a key role during the progression of HF in patients with low T3 syndrome.[24–32]

Up to 30% of patients with HF have low serum T_3 levels; they are associated with CV changes in humans. Although the α-MHC isoform is prevalently expressed in the human heart, changes in the MHC isoform expression can occur in the human atria in patients with congestive HF and in severe hypothyroidism.[33,34] These changes also are linked to a decreased expression of SERCA 2 and increased cytoskeletal abnormalities, with consequent modifications in contractility, wall stress, chamber diameters, and wall thickness.[34]

Studies in humans have demonstrated that low serum T_3 levels correlate with the severity of HF when assessed by the New York Heart Association (NYHA) classification.[35–37] Low T3

Table 1
Main findings in heart failure and effects of low T_3 syndrome on the cardiovascular system

	Heart Failure	Heart Failure + Low T3 Syndrome
LV systolic function	↓	↓↓
LV diastolic function	↓	↓↓
SVR	↑	↑↑
Cardiac contractility	↓	↓↓
Renal function	↓	↓↓
CO	↓	↓↓
Alterations in the myocyte shape	↑	↑↑

syndrome occurs with a higher incidence in patients with NYHA classes III and IV compared with NHYA I and NYHA II.[34–37] In addition, the negative prognostic role of the low T3 is enhanced in patients with higher BNP concentration, both in acute decompensated HF and chronic compensated HF.[37] The abnormal TH pattern in patients with HF is associated with a high incidence of fatal events. In a large cohort of cardiac patients with ischemic HF and nonischemic HF, T3 levels and left ventricular ejection fraction (LVEF) were the only independent predictive variables of both cardiac and cumulative deaths at multivariate analysis.[36] Patients with low T3 levels and reduced LVEF had the highest mortality compared with patients with similar LVEF but normal T3 levels.[36] These results suggest that T3 levels can be useful to identify patients at high risk for death.

TREATMENT WITH THYROID HORMONES

Hypothyroid cardiac alterations in the failing heart can be reversible with TH replacement therapy. The T3 supplementation in the culture of neonatal cardiomyocytes was associated with a positive change in the myocyte shape, with an increased ratio of the major to minor cell axis and an increase in the synthesis of α-MHC.[38–41] Treatment with physiologic doses of T3 also normalized the SERCA2 contents of cardyomyocytes, improving systolic and diastolic functions and heart performance.[38–41]

This Opinion is supported by the Following consideration: (1) the evidence that T3 has positive effects on the CV function, (2) the observation that even mild TH deficiency is associated with a worse outcome in cardiac patients, (3) the negative prognostic impact of the low T3 syndrome, and (4) the improvement of the cardiac dysfunction after TH administration. On this basis, LT4, LT3, and TH analogs have been administered to improve the prognosis of patients with HF.

Some studies used LT4 in patients with HF or dilated cardiomyopathy. Moruzzi and colleagues[42,43] performed 2 randomized placebo-controlled studies to evaluate the short-term and long-term CV effects of oral LT4 at a dose of 0.1 mg per day. In both of these studies, LT4 was able to significantly improve cardiac contractility, resting LVEF, CO, and exercise capacity.[42,43] Similar results were observed by Malik and colleagues,[44] who administered intravenous LT4 (20 μg/h) in 10 consecutive patients with severe systolic HF, which progressed to cardiogenic shock. These patients had a significant improvement in cardiac index, pulmonary capillary wedge pressure, and mean arterial pressure after 24 hours and 36 hours of LT4 administration.

The first study that used LT3 was performed by Hamilton and colleagues.[45] In a small nonrandomized trial, these investigators used an intravenous bolus of liothyronine (LT3) followed by LT3 infusion in patients with advanced HF and low T3 syndrome.[45] CO improved significantly 2 hours after T3 administration. Moreover, SVR significantly decreased without considerable changes in blood pressure. Comparable findings were observed by Pingitore and coworkers.[46,47] They administered physiologic doses of LT3 (20 μg/d/m^2 body surface) for a period of 96 hours in 6 patients with advanced HF and low T3 syndrome.[46] A progressive reduction in SVR, an increase in LVEF, and an improvement of CO were observed after T3 administration. These positive results were confirmed in a placebo-controlled study by the same investigators.[47] They administered a 3-day LT3 infusion in patients with chronic and stable dilated cardiomyopathy and low T3 syndrome. Their results showed an improved cardiac performance and an increase in total cardiac work, which were associated with a concomitant improvement of the neuroendocrine pattern (decreased noradrenaline plasma levels and N-terminal prohormone of BNP).[47]

All these studies demonstrated that THs were well tolerated with no occurrence of major or minor side effects and without any increase in atrial arrhythmias or heart rate.

THYROID HORMONE ANALOGS IN HEART FAILURE

3,5-diiodothyropropionic acid (DITPA), a TH analog with a cardiac inotropic selectivity, was tested in humans to treat congestive HF in a randomized clinical trial.[48] DITPA was able to improve cardiac index and diastolic function and decrease SVR; it also improved total cholesterol and LDL cholesterol values and triglycerides. Its use, however, was not associated with an improvement of CHF symptoms and generally was poorly tolerated by the patients because of an average weight loss of 11 kg. This decrease in weight was not related to the gastrointestinal side effects, which were common in patients treated with DITPA.[48] DITPA also suppressed the hypothalamic-pituitary-thyroid axis and had a negative effect on bone by increasing bone turnover.[48] Unfortunately, these several adverse events caused the withdrawal of DITPA from clinical trials.

SUMMARY

Large prospective multicenter studies are needed to assess the usefulness of THs in treating and/or preventing the evolution of HF. Further research is needed to establish which drugs (T3, T4, or analogs) could be useful in treating patients with HF. The timing of TH administration and the best schedule for therapy (their dosage and route of administration intravenous or orally) also should be assessed.

REFERENCES

1. Biondi B, Palmieri EA, Lombardi G, et al. Effects of thyroid hormone on cardiac function: the relative importance of heart rate, loading conditions, and myocardial contractility in the regulation of cardiac performance in human hyperthyroidism. J Clin Endocrinol Metab 2002;87(3):968–74.

2. Cooper DS, Biondi B. Subclinical thyroid disease. Lancet 2012;379:1142–54.

3. Biondi B, Cooper DS. The clinical significance of subclinical thyroid dysfunction. Endocr Rev 2008; 29:76–131.

4. Klein I, Biondi B. Endocrine disorders and cardiovascular disease. In: Zipes DP, Libby P, Bonow RO, et al, editors. Braunwald's heart disease: a Textbook of cardiovascular Medicine. 11th edition. Elsevier; 2018 [Chapter 92] 92-1- 92-14. ISBN 9780323555920.

5. Razvi S, Jabbar A, Pingitore A, et al. Thyroid hormones and cardiovascular function and diseases. J Am Coll Cardiol 2018;71(16):1781–96.

6. Bassett JH, Harvey CB, Williams GR. Mechanisms of thyroid hormone receptor–specific nuclear and extra nuclear actions. Mol Cell Endocrinol 2003; 213:1.

7. Fazio S, Palmieri EA, Lombardi G, et al. Effects of thyroid hormone on the cardiovascular system. Recent Prog Horm Res 2004;59:31–50.

8. Biondi B, Klein I. Hypothyroidism as a risk factor for cardiovascular disease. Endocrine 2004;24(1):1–13.

9. Biondi B, Palmieri EA, Lombardi G, et al. Subclinical thyroid dysfunction and the heart. Ann Intern Med 2003;134:904–14.

10. Biondi B, Palmieri EA, Lombardi G, et al. Subclinical hypothyroidism and cardiac function. Thyroid 2002; 12:505–10.

11. Biondi B, Fazio S, Palmieri EA, et al. Left ventricular diastolic dysfunction in patients with subclinical hypothyroidism. J Clin Endocrinol Metab 1999;84:2064–7.

12. Ripoli A, Pingitore A, Favilli B, et al. Does subclinical hypothyroidism affect cardiac pump performance? Evidence from a magnetic resonance imaging study. J Am Coll Cardiol 2005;45:439–45.

13. Biondi B. Mechanisms in endocrinology: Heart failure and thyroid dysfunction. Eur J Endocrinol 2012;167:609–18.

14. Gencer B, Collet TH, Virgini V, et al. Subclinical thyroid dysfunction and the risk of heart failure events: an individual participant data analysis from 6 prospective cohorts. Circulation 2012;126:1040–9.

15. Iervasi G, Molinaro S, Landi P, et al. Association between increased mortality and mild thyroid dysfunction in cardiac patients. Arch Intern Med 2007;167: 1526–32.

16. Biondi B. Natural history, diagnosis and management of subclinical thyroid dysfunction. Best Pract Res Clin Endocrinol Metab 2012;26:431–46.

17. Biondi B, Wartofsky L. Treatment with thyroid hormone. Endocr Rev 2014;35(3):433–512.

18. Garber JR, Cobin RH, Gharib H, et al. Clinical practice guidelines for hypothyroidism in adults: cosponsored by the American Association of Clinical Endocrinologists and the American Thyroid Association. Thyroid 2012;22:1200–35.

19. Fliers E, Bianco AC, Langouche L, et al. Thyroid function in critically ill patients. Lancet Diabetes Endocrinol 2015;3:816–25.

20. Van den Berghe G. Non-thyroidal illness in the ICU: a syndrome with different faces. Thyroid 2014;24: 1456–65.

21. De Groot LJ. Dangerous dogmas in medicine: the nonthyroidal illness syndrome. J Clin Endocrinol Metab 1999;84:151–64.

22. Gereben B, Zavacki AM, Ribich S, et al. Cellular and molecular basis of deiodinase-regulated thyroid hormone signaling. Endocr Rev 2008;29: 898–938.

23. Braunwals E. Heart failure. JACC Heart Fail 2013; 1(1):1–20.

24. Diano S, Horvath TL. Type 3 deiodinase in hypoxia: to cool or to kill? Cell Metab 2008;7:363–4.

25. Wassen FW, Schiel AE, Kuiper GG, et al. Induction of thyroid hormone-degrading deiodinase in cardiac hypertrophy and failure. Endocrinology 2002;143: 2812–5.

26. Pol CJ, Muller A, Zuidwijk MJ, et al. Left-ventricular remodeling after myocardial infarction is associated with a cardiomyocyte-specific hypothyroid condition. Endocrinology 2011;152:669–79.

27. Katzeff HL, Powell SR, Ojamaa K. Alterations in cardiac contractility and gene expression during low-T3 syndrome: prevention with T3. Am J Physiol 1997; 273:E951–6.

28. Forini F, Paolicchi A, Pizzorusso T, et al. 3, 5, 30-Triiodothyronine deprivation affects phenotype and intracellular [Ca2] of human cardiomyocytes in culture. Cardiovasc Res 2001;51:322–30.

29. Liu Z, Gerdes AM. Influence of hypothyroidism and the reversal of hypothyroidism on hemodynamics and cell size in the adult rat heart. J Mol Cell Cardiol 1990;22:1339–48.

30. Kinugawa K, Yonekura K, Ribeiro RC, et al. Regulation of thyroid hormone receptor isoforms in physiological and pathological cardiac hypertrophy. Circ Res 2001;89:591–8.

31. Rajagopalan V, Gerdes AM. Role of thyroid hormones in ventricular remodeling. Curr Heart Fail Rep 2015;12:141–9.

32. Cokkinos DV, Chryssanthopoulos S. Thyroid hormones and cardiac remodeling. Heart Fail Rev 2016;21:365–72.

33. Ladenson PW, Sherman SI, Baughman KL, et al. Reversible alterations in myocardial gene expression in a young man with dilated cardiomyopathy and hypothyroidism. Proc Natl Acad Sci U S A 1992;89:5251–5.

34. Razeghi P, Young ME, Alcorn JL, et al. Metabolic gene expression in fetal and failing human heart. Circulation 2001;104:2923–31.

35. Iervasi G, Pingitore A, Landi P, et al. Low-T3 syndrome: a strong prognostic predictor of death in patients with heart disease. Circulation 2003;107:708–13.

36. Pingitore A, Landi P, Taddei MC, et al. Triiodothyronine levels for risk stratification of patients with chronic heart failure. Am J Med 2005;118:132–6.

37. Passino C, Pingitore A, Landi P, et al. Prognostic value of combined measurement of brain natriuretic peptide and triiodothyronine in heart failure. J Card Fail 2009;15:35–40.

38. Pantos C, Dritsas A, Mourouzis I, et al. Thyroid hormone is a critical determinant of myocardial performance in patients with heart failure: potential therapeutic implications. Eur J Endocrinol 2007;157:515–20.

39. Schmidt-Ott UM, Ascheim DD. Thyroid hormone and heart failure. Curr Heart Fail Rep 2006;3:114–9.

40. Gerdes AM, Iervasi G. Thyroid replacement therapy and heart failure. Circulation 2010;122:385–93.

41. Gerdes AM. Restoration of thyroid hormone balance: a game changer in the treatment of heart failure? Am J Physiol Heart Circ Physiol 2015;308:H1–10.

42. Moruzzi P, Doria E, Agostoni PG, et al. Usefulness of L-thyroxine to improve cardiac and exercise performance in idiopathic dilated cardiomyopathy. Am J Cardiol 1994;73:374–8.

43. Moruzzi P, Doria E, Agostoni PG. Medium-term effectiveness of L-thyroxine treatment in idiopathic dilated cardiomyopathy. Am J Med 1996;101:461–7.

44. Malik FS, Mehra MR, Uber PA, et al. Intravenous thyroid hormone supplementation in heart failure with cardiogenic shock. J Card Fail 1999;5:31–7.

45. Hamilton MA, Stevenson LW, Fonarow GC, et al. Safety and hemodynamic effects of intravenous triiodothyronine in advanced congestive heart failure. Am J Cardiol 1998;81:443–7.

46. Pingitore A, Iervasi G. Triiodothyronine (T3) effects on cardiovascular system in patients with heart failure. Recent Pat Cardiovasc Drug Discov 2008;3:19–27.

47. Pingitore A, Galli E, Barison A, et al. Acute effects of triiodothyronine (T3) replacement therapy in patients with chronic heart failure and low-T3 syndrome: a randomized, placebo-controlled study. J Clin Endocrinol Metab 2008;93:1351–8.

48. Goldman S, McCarren M, Morkin E, et al. DITPA (3,5-diiodothyropropionic acid), a thyroid hormone analog to treat heart failure: phase II trial veterans affairs cooperative study. Circulation 2009;119:3093–100.

Acromegaly and Heart Failure

Annamaria Colao, MD, PhD[a],*, Ludovica F.S. Grasso, MD[a], Carolina Di Somma, MD, PhD[b], Rosario Pivonello, MD, PhD[a]

KEYWORDS

• Acromegaly • Pituitary adenoma • Cardiomyopathy • Heart failure • Medical therapy

KEY POINTS

- Cardiovascular disease represents the most frequent comorbidity and represents one of the most important cause of death in acromegaly.
- Acromegaly is associated with a typical cardiomyopathy, characterized by biventricular hypertrophy, mainly involving the left ventricle, in 80%, and consequent diastolic dysfunction, in up to 58% of patients with active disease.
- The progression to systolic dysfunction is generally uncommon, and observed in less than 3% of patients. Consequently, the presence of overt congestive heart failure (CHF) is rare in acromegaly, ranging between 1% and 4%, in patients with untreated and uncontrolled disease.
- Control of acromegaly, induced by either pituitary surgery or medical therapy, improves cardiac structure and performance. Overall, the 1- and 5-year mortality (or transplantation) rates for patients with chronic symptomatic CHF were 25% and 37.5%, respectively.

INTRODUCTION

Growth hormone (GH) is principally involved in the regulation of somatic growth, including cardiac development and function, and exerts its effects either directly or indirectly by stimulating the production of its tissue effector insulin-like growth factor-1 (IGF-I), which ultimately mediates GH actions on peripheral tissues.[1–4] In particular, GH/IGF-I axis plays an important role in cardiac growth, myocardial contractility, and vascular system.[3] Abnormalities of the GH/IGF-I axis contribute in determining cardiovascular disease, as suggested by clinical studies reporting an increased risk for cardiovascular morbidity and mortality in GH deficiency (GHD) and GH excess.[1–6]

Acromegaly represents a clinical condition characterized by GH excess. It is a progressive disease resulting from the increased GH and, consequently, IGF-I levels, caused by, in most cases, a GH-secreting pituitary adenoma.[1] The prolonged exposure to GH excess induces progressive somatic alterations and a wide range of systemic manifestations, mainly including cardiovascular, respiratory, and metabolic complications.[1,2] Cardiovascular disease represents the most prevalent comorbidity, accounting for up to 80% of complications in patients with acromegaly, and has historically reported to contribute to nearly 50% of deaths.[7] However, recent studies demonstrated that the most common cause of mortality in acromegaly is cancer, followed by cardiovascular disease.[8,9] Therefore, nowadays, cardiovascular disease represents the most frequent comorbidity and still represents one of the most important causes of death in acromegaly.[2,7–9] Arterial hypertension and heart disease constitute the major negative survival determinants in acromegaly, whereas overt congestive heart failure (CHF) is one of the poor prognostic sign of acromegaly.[1]

Because data on cardiac failure in acromegaly are extremely limited, in the present review we

Disclosure: The authors have nothing to disclose.
[a] Dipartimento di Medicina Clinica e Chirurgia, Sezione di Endocrinologia, University Federico II, Naples, Italy;
[b] IRCCS SDN, Napoli Via Gianturco 113, Naples 80143, Italy
* Corresponding author. University Federico II, Via S. Pansini 5, Naples 80131, Italy.
E-mail address: colao@unina.it

heartfailure.theclinics.com

discuss the cardiovascular implication of GH excess and the evolution process of acromegaly cardiomyopathy to CHF.

PHYSIOLOGIC EFFECTS OF GROWTH HORMONE AND INSULIN-LIKE GROWTH FACTOR-I ON CARDIOVASCULAR SYSTEM

The relationship between GH/IGF-I axis and cardiovascular system has been demonstrated by several experimental studies.[5,10] In physiologic conditions, GH/IGF-I axis exerts relevant cardiovascular actions aimed to regulate cardiac growth and myocardial contractility, thus contributing to the maintenance of cardiac mass and function in normal adults (**Fig. 1**).[5] Functional receptors for GH and IGF-I are also expressed in blood vessels.[11] Thus GH/IGF-I axis interacts specifically with the vascular system, regulating the vascular tone and the peripheral resistance,[4] which indirectly affects cardiac performance.[6] In addition, GH up-regulates the myocardial expression of IGF-I mRNA.[11] Besides direct actions of GH, endocrine or autocrine/paracrine effects of locally produced IGF-I on the cardiovascular system are likely operating as well, making it difficult to differentiate between the direct effects of GH and those IGF-I-mediated.[12]

GH and IGF-I receptors expressed in cardiomyocytes are responsible for direct actions of both hormones on cardiac growth and metabolism. However, most of the studies have failed to show direct, IGF-I-independent hypertrophic effects of GH on cardiomyocytes.[5] In contrast, experimental models clearly demonstrated that IGF-I per se causes hypertrophy of cultured rat cardiomyocytes.[13] The increased cardiac protein synthesis is mainly mediated by the activation of the phosphatidylinositol 3-kinase (PI3K) eAkt pathway,[14] one of the two major pathways of IGF-I signaling,[15] and by delaying cardiomyocyte apoptosis.[15] GH and IGF-I also have direct effects on myocardial contractility and cardiac output in humans and experimental animals. These effects are mediated by the increased mRNA expression for specific muscle proteins, including troponin, myosin light chain-2, and a-actin.[5,6,10] GH promotes the shift toward the V3 myosin isoform with lower ATPase activity, which may decrease the energy demand of the contractile process.[5,10,16] In addition, GH and IGF-I increase intracellular calcium content and calcium sensitivity of myofilaments in cardiomyocytes.[5,16] The endothelial cells have high-affinity binding sites for IGF-I. In particular, the local production of IGF-I causes endothelial-dependent vasodilatation via the stimulation of the nitric oxide production.[5] Moreover, IGF-I may cause vasodilatation through nonendothelium-dependent actions, by increasing the activity of the Naþ, Kþ-ATPase in vascular smooth muscle cells,[17] with possible contribution of increased gene expression of the vascular smooth muscle ATP-sensitive potassium channels.[4]

Growth Hormone and Insulin-Like Growth Factor-I in Cardiac Heart Failure

CHF is a complex syndrome with hemodynamic impairment characterized by inadequate blood

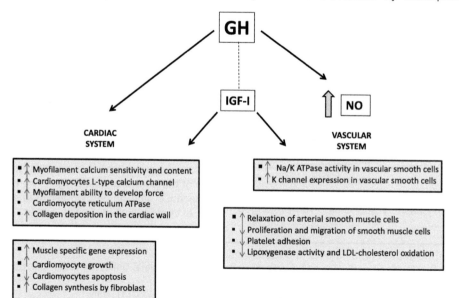

Fig. 1. Physiologic effects of GH and IGF-I on the cardiovascular system. LDL, low-density lipoprotein; NO, nitric oxide.

supply to peripheral tissues.[10,18] CHF is a progressive disorder in which a complex interaction of hemodynamic, neurohormonal, and metabolic disturbances leads to subsequent immune activation. The greatest attention has been given to the concept that the progression of CHF is caused by neurohormonal abnormalities and this has led to substantial therapeutic benefits for CHF.[10,18] In particular, many studies reported reduced IGF-I levels in the CHF population and the beneficial effect of GH therapy in improving CHF.[10,18–24] Low levels of IGF-I seems to correlate with the degree of systolic dysfunction, the presence of cachexia and skeletal muscle weakness, and indices of neurohormonal and cytokine activation.[21] These data support the concept that low IGF-I in CHF is not a simple biomarker, but it is also mechanistically linked to CHF and its severity.[10,25] In particular, GH secretion was assessed by combined GHRH plus arginine stimulatory test in patients with CHF compared with control subjects, showing that patients with CHF reported a markedly impaired GH response, with a prevalence of 30% to 40% of GHD.[22–24] The systemic hemodynamic impairment caused by CHF can significantly alter local homeostasis in the pituitary vasculature, through stasis in vein drainage and/or suboptimal arterial supply in anterior hypophysis, with subsequent GHD. However, no direct evidence using imaging techniques supports this hypothesis.[10,25] Even though this is a reasonable explanation for the occurrence of GHD in about one-third of CHF population, additional factors can include background therapy for CHF (ie, angiotensin-converting enzyme-I and digitalis interfere with IGF-I levels), chronic systemic inflammation, and primary or CHF-related hypothalamus damage.[10] Catabolic and inflammatory conditions physiologically induce a dramatic decrease in IGF-I levels, and it is well known that CHF is characterized by low-grade systemic inflammation and cytokine activation, which may consequently lower IGF-I circulating levels.[26] However, no systematic evaluation has been so far conducted to deeply investigate these alterations in patients with CHF.

CHF is a progressive disorder; at the initial stage in most cases patients remain asymptomatic or minimally symptomatic, after the initial decline in pumping capacity of the heart. To preserve cardiac output, compensatory mechanisms are activated, including the adrenergic nervous system and salt- and water-retaining systems.[18] When compensatory mechanisms become unable to prevent elevation of left ventricular (LV) diastolic filling pressures and/or reduction of cardiac output, patients become symptomatic, resulting in an increased morbidity and mortality.[18] Few studies speculated that alterations of the GH/IGF-I axis also have a time-course intimately related to the stage and severity of CHF.[22,27,28] It was hypothesized that in the initial stage of CHF, IGF-I values are normal or slightly elevated probably trying to reduce inotropism and proapoptotic signaling typical of the CHF syndrome. In the intermediate stage, IGF-I levels tend to decrease probably because of insufficient hepatic IGF-I generation. In advanced stages of CHF, GH resistance sets in, leading to reduced IGF-I and markedly increased GH circulating levels.[10] No study has systematically investigated a relationship between severity of CHF and IGF-I levels and no definitive evidence is available on the prognostic value of GH/IGF-I axis alterations, because data are still controversial. However, several clinical studies have been performed to evaluate the effects of adjunctive GH therapy in patients with CHF.[22,29–37] Some studies suggest that GH treatment increases LV ejection fraction and reduces systemic vascular resistance in patients with CHF but results are contradictory.[10,22,25]

ACROMEGALIC CARDIOMYOPATHY AND HEART FAILURE

Acromegaly is associated with a typical cardiomyopathy, characterized by biventricular hypertrophy, mainly involving the LV in 80%, and consequent diastolic dysfunction in 44% of patients with active disease.[1,2,7,38,39] Additional relevant cardiovascular complications are represented by arterial hypertension, valvulopathies, arrhythmias, and vascular endothelial dysfunction, which, together with the respiratory and metabolic complications, contribute to the development of cardiac disease and the increased cardiovascular risk in acromegaly.[1,7] The pathogenesis of acromegalic cardiomyopathy includes a direct action of GH and IGF-I excess on the heart, and an indirect mechanisms by which GH and IGF-I excess induces arterial hypertension and disorders of lipid and glucose metabolism, resulting in cardiac glucotoxicity and lipotoxicity and cardiac hypertrophy and remodeling.[40] The pathogenesis of acromegalic cardiomyopathy develops after three steps (**Fig. 2**).[1] The early phase is reversible and is characterized by initial cardiac hypertrophy, with increase of heart rate and systolic output, configuring the hyperkinetic syndrome.[1,41] In the middle phase of untreated or uncontrolled disease, cardiac hypertrophy becomes more evident, with signs of diastolic dysfunction and the appearance of systolic dysfunction on effort.[1] In the end-stage of

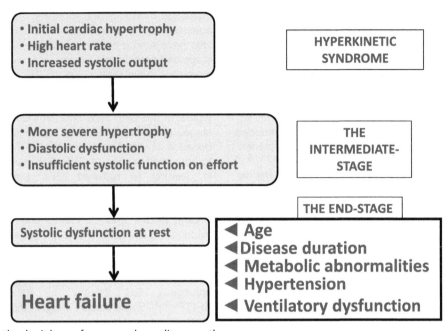

Fig. 2. Pathophysiology of acromegaly cardiomyopathy.

untreated or uncontrolled disease, cardiac damage may include systolic dysfunction at rest and CHF, until the development of dilative cardiomyopathy, which is not reversible even with the treatment of the acromegaly.[1,7] GH excess exerts different and apparently opposite effects on the heart, enhancing cardiac performance in the early stage and causing cardiac dysfunction in the end-stage. The precise mechanisms by which short-term GH excess displays overall beneficial effects on cardiovascular performance, and long-term exposure induces cardiac dysfunction and progression to CHF, is still unknown and seems to be linked to the development of myocardial fibrosis and inflammation.[10,42]

At diagnosis, cardiac hypertrophy is a common feature in patients with acromegaly, in particular in those with a long duration of disease.[43] Acromegalic heart has thickened walls but rarely the cardiac chambers are enlarged.[1] At histology, interstitial fibrosis, myofibrillar derangement, increased extracellular collagen deposition, and areas of monocyte necrosis and lymphomononuclear infiltration are the most relevant abnormalities, progressively impairing the whole organ architecture.[44,45] Different echocardiographic studies have confirmed these histologic findings, reporting cardiac fibrosis to be common in the acromegalic heart.[45] However, more recent studies have found cardiac fibrosis to be totally absent[46] or rare[47] in patients with active acromegaly when evaluated by cardiac MRI (CMRI). Coexistence of cardiovascular comorbidities,

including arterial hypertension, arrhythmias, and valvulopathy, together with vascular endothelial dysfunction and disorders of glucose and lipid metabolism, may worsen cardiomyopathy.[48] Earlier studies using conventional echocardiography had estimated that 11% to 78% of patients with acromegaly have LV hypertrophy[2,46,49–53]; however, more recent studies using CMRI, which is the gold standard for evaluating LV hypertrophy and fibrosis, have found a much lower prevalence.[47,54,55] In particular, a recent study detected LV hypertrophy in 5% and 31% of patients when analyzed respectively by CMRI and echocardiographic studies,[47] suggesting that echocardiographic studies methodology may overestimate LV hypertrophy presence in patients with acromegaly. Therefore, LV hypertrophy frequency in contemporary cohorts of patients with acromegaly seems to be lower than the frequency observed in previous studies. This could be caused in part by earlier diagnosis, technical differences between echocardiographic studies and CMRI, and more effective agents to control acromegaly.

The main functional disturbance in acromegalic cardiomyopathy is the diastolic dysfunction, characterized by an inadequate filling capacity.[7] Although diastolic dysfunction is frequently observed in 11% to 58% of patients, it is usually mild, without clinical consequence. The progression to systolic dysfunction is generally uncommon,[56,57] not seen or observed in less than 3% of patients in most recent studies,[2,50,56,57] particularly in the end-stage of acromegalic cardiomyopathy in patients with untreated or uncontrolled disease.[7] The relative risk to develop systolic dysfunction seems to be higher in patients with acromegaly compared with control subjects,[50] suggesting a potential cumulative effect of the exposure to chronic GH/IGF-I excess.

Because overt systolic dysfunction is not common, some studies aimed to evaluate the presence of incipient myocardial damage,[58,59] evaluating myocardial strain, which consider the deformation of the myocardial fibers during systole (calculated as the percent change in the myocardial fiber length between the end-diastole and the end-systole[60]). The impairment in global longitudinal strain, a marker of subclinical systolic dysfunction,[2] has been studied in patients with acromegaly and data are so far controversial.[58,59] In a previous study by Di Bello and colleagues[59] including 22 patients with active acromegaly and 25 control subjects, myocardial systolic strain and strain rate values, indices of regional systolic heart deformation, were lower in patients with acromegaly compared with control subjects, which may indicate subclinical systolic dysfunction. However, a recent studies by Volschan and colleagues[58] evaluated the presence of myocardial strain in 37 patients with active acromegaly and 48 controls using a speckle tracking echocardiography, a technique that represents a more accurate method quantifying regional and global strain.[61] In this study no difference in myocardial systolic strain between patients and control subjects was reported, suggesting that patients with acromegaly have a low chance of evolution to systolic dysfunction and agrees with recent studies that show a lower frequency of cardiac disease in these patients.[58]

Consequently, the presence of overt CHF is uncommon in acromegaly, ranging between 1% and 4%.[2,10,56,62] In a recent multicenter French study that included 943 patients, CHF was present in only 1.9% of patients at diagnosis.[56] In contrast, in a Danish national study, CHF was increased in patients with acromegaly compared with control subjects (hazard ratio, 2.5 [1.4–4.5]), and the risk was more pronounced in the 3-year period before diagnosis.[62] In this latter study, CHF prevalence was lower than previously reported: older studies, however, were performed when the treatment of acromegaly (and its comorbidities) was less aggressive and when CHF was diagnosed based on less modern criteria and/or without the use of echocardiography.[57] In addition, the treatment and follow-up of patients with acromegaly is significantly improved, markedly during the last two decades, and the risk of CHF is probably lower than before.[57] A recent study by Petrossians and colleagues,[38] including 3171 patients with acromegaly from The Liège Acromegaly Survey, observed cardiac hypertrophy in 15.5% of patients at diagnosis and CHF in 1.6%. Patients with cardiac hypertrophy and CHF at diagnosis were significantly older at diagnosis (6–13 years) than those without these cardiovascular complications. In this situation, it becomes difficult to attribute a causative role for GH hypersecretion to cardiac morbidities in acromegaly, and as patients age, the presence of acromegaly may simply represent one of the many contributory risk factors.[38] No specific risk factors for developing CHF were found in acromegalic patients.

In contrast, no increased prevalence of coronary artery disease was found in patients with newly diagnosed acromegaly.[63,64] Similarly, the extent of carotid atherosclerosis and carotic internal media thickening in patients with acromegaly was not higher than that in subjects without acromegaly.[63,65] The reasons for this unexpected observation are still unclear, but this finding suggests that the known atherogenic effects of hypertension, insulin resistance, and diabetes induced by GH excess[66] are counterbalanced by cardioprotective factors.[64]

Several biomarkers have been identified to be associated with atherosclerotic morbidity and are used in clinical practice to determine individual cardiovascular risk and treatment strategy. Among these markers, the inflammatory protein high-sensitive C-reactive protein (hs-CRP) is related to cardiovascular disease and is stimulated by the proinflammatory cytokine interleukin 6, and the N-terminal probrain natriuretic peptide (NT-proBNP) is used as a diagnostic parameter for CHF.[67] Different studies have evaluated whether acromegaly might be related to changes in hs-CRP and NT-proBNP and data are contradictory.[68] Lower than normal values of hs-CRP have been shown in most studies on patients with active acromegaly,[66,68–72] but not all studies.[73] Data on NT-proBNP are contradictory, in particular, some studies reported low levels in active acromegaly,[68,70,74] whereas others reported that NT-proBNP levels seems to be not influenced by the acromegaly status.[73,75] A recent study by Verhelst and colleagues[68] evaluated hs-CRP and NT-proBNP in 200 patients from the Belgian acromegaly registry, comparing these data with those obtained from a reference population. Patients with active acromegaly had significantly lower values of NT-proBNP and hs-CRP compared with patients with controlled disease, and even lower values of hs-CRP compared with control subjects.[68] In controlled acromegaly, hs-CRP was comparable with those of the normal population, whereas NT-proBNP was higher.[68] The low value of hs-CRP might be linked to the low incidence of coronary artery disease in these patients,[63,64] despite the increase in other cardiovascular risk factors, such as arterial hypertension or diabetes. It remains unclear if the low levels of NT-proBNP reported in active acromegaly reflect a beneficial effect on the heart or not. BNP and its prohormone proBNP are secreted by the heart in response to volume overload and induce natriuresis, predicting all-cause mortality and cardiovascular events including CHF.[67] Although low levels of this cardiac marker are considered advantageous for the heart in the general population, it is unclear if this is also applicable in acromegaly. Moreover, a direct inhibition of BNP or NT-proBNP by GH, independent from cardiac function, cannot be excluded in these patients.[68]

EFFECTS OF ACROMEGALY THERAPIES ON CARDIOMYOPATHY AND HEART FAILURE

The acromegaly therapy has significantly evolved over the last two decades, with less frequent use of radiotherapy and the introduction of new pharmacologic treatments.[76–79] The optimal management of acromegaly resulted in a normalized mortality rate of these patients compared with general population, and a change in the prognosis of different acromegaly complications.[76,80]

The therapeutic goal in acromegaly is to restore normal GH and IGF-I secretion; remove or reduce the pituitary tumor; preserve the normal residual pituitary function; prevent recurrences; improve comorbidities, which contribute to the unfavorable long-term outcome; and reduce the mortality.[76] The approaches to therapy for acromegaly include pituitary surgery, radiotherapy; and medical therapy; these latter include somatostatin analogues (SSA), dopamine-agonists, and the GH-receptor antagonist pegvisomant (PEG). Control of acromegaly, induced by either pituitary surgery or medical therapy, improves cardiac structure and performance.[7,39]

In particular, in patients receiving SSA, LV hypertrophy rapidly reduces following hormone normalization,[51,81–84] and the improvement in diastolic and systolic dysfunction occurs in those achieving hormone excess control.[85] Persistence of uncontrolled acromegaly is associated with further impairment of cardiac performance.[85] However, the recovery of LV hypertrophy or diastolic and systolic dysfunction depends not only on the correction of hormone excess but also on patient age,[64,86] disease duration,[64,81] and the control of metabolic comorbidities.[81] In fact, the achievement of disease control induced by 12-month SSA treatment has been shown to normalize LV mass in 100% of young and in 50% of middle-aged patients,[81] and ejection fraction response at peak exercise in 80% of young and in 50% of middle-aged patients.[81] A similar effect of SSA and surgery has been demonstrated to improve LV hypertrophy and diastolic function, whereas systolic function was more evidently improved in patients treated with SSA than in patients treated by surgery.[86] Five years treatment with SSA, as first-line therapy, induced a significant improvement in the prevalence of LV hypertrophy, diastolic and systolic dysfunction, arterial hypertension, arrhythmias, and lipid profile,[82] and a slight decrease in the prevalence of the impairment of glucose metabolism.[51] In patients resistant to SSA, long-term PEG monotherapy has been demonstrated to improve acromegalic cardiomyopathy, by decreasing cardiac hypertrophy and enhancing diastolic and systolic function.[87] Recent evidence has also demonstrated that combined therapy with SSA and PEG exerts a beneficial effect on acromegalic cardiomyopathy,[88] improving cardiac mass and diastolic function.[88] Until now, no studies have described the effects of cabergoline on cardiovascular complications in acromegaly.[2]

A study conducted by Rajasoorya and colleagues[89] found that the patient's life expectancy was predicted to be less than 15 years when systolic dysfunction was diagnosed. Bihan and colleagues[57] studied retrospectively 10 patients with both acromegaly and CHF. CHF was diagnosed before, concomitantly, or after acromegaly in two, five, and two patients, respectively. Three patients were referred with terminal CHF requiring transplantation. One patient had transient CHF associated with a hypertensive crisis. The other eight patients had symptomatic chronic CHF. Disease control was achieved in five patients, reporting a long-term survival of 2 to 16 years from CHF diagnosis. Three patients reported a partial or a failure of disease control and died at 1 and 5 years. Overall, the 1- and 5-year mortality (or transplantation) rates for patients with chronic symptomatic CHF were 25% and 37.5%, respectively.[57]

At the end-stage of acromegaly cardiomyopathy, when CHF occurred until the development of dilative cardiomyopathy, it is generally not reversible, despite the treatment of acromegaly.[7]

Moreover, also cardiovascular complications, including LV hypertrophy,[86] may persist even after the achievement of disease control, particularly in 50% of middle-age patients and long disease duration.[81] Therefore early diagnosis and prompt treatment of hormone excess is crucial in the management of acromegaly, monitoring regularly cardiac structure and function, even in patients cured from acromegaly, particularly in elderly patients and those with long-term uncontrolled disease.

SUMMARY

Active acromegaly is associated with an increased mortality compared with the general population, with cardiovascular diseases representing one of the most important causes of death. However, despite the increased mortality related to cardiovascular disease, CHF is generally uncommon in these patients, being reported in 1% to 4% patients. This low prevalence, confirmed in recent studies, should be caused by an improved management of these patients and a possible protective role of GH excess on the heart.

Early diagnosis and prompt treatment are the best way to limit the progression of acromegaly cardiomyopathy. Appropriate and effective treatment of acromegaly should be started early to obtain strict hormone control since beneficial effects on cardiovascular comorbidities and mortality have been reported in patients achieving disease control. In particular, stringent control of hormone excess is associated with significant improvement in cardiac hypertrophy, and diastolic and systolic function, demonstrating that biochemical control leads to an overall improvement in cardiac structure and performance in patients with acromegaly. However, monitoring cardiovascular disease is crucial in elderly patients with long disease duration, despite the achievement of disease control, to control and prevent the progression of acromegaly cardiomyopathy to CHF. Close dialogue among endocrinologists and cardiologists involved in the management of patients with acromegaly is of extreme importance for the optimal care of these patients.

Further studies are needed to better understand the possible presence of cardioprotective factors in acromegaly.

REFERENCES

1. Colao A, Ferone D, Marzullo P, et al. Systemic complications of acromegaly: epidemiology, pathogenesis, and management. Endocr Rev 2004;25: 102–52.
2. Gadelha MR, Kasuki L, Lim DST, et al. Systemic complications of acromegaly and the impact of the current treatment landscape: an update. Endocr Rev 2019;40(1):268–332.
3. Colao A, Di Somma C, Savanelli MC, et al. Beginning to end: cardiovascular implications of growth hormone (GH) deficiency and GH therapy. Growth Horm IGF Res 2006;16:S41–8.
4. Colao A. The GH-IGF-I axis and the cardiovascular system: clinical implications. Clin Endocrinol 2008; 69(3):347–58.
5. Isgaard J, Arcopinto M, Karason K, et al. GH and the cardiovascular system: an update on a topic at heart. Endocrine 2015;48(1):25–35.
6. Di Somma C, Scarano E, Savastano S, et al. Cardiovascular alterations in adult GH deficiency. Best Pract Res Clin Endocrinol Metab 2017;31(1):25–34.
7. Pivonello R, Auriemma RS, Grasso LF, et al. Complications of acromegaly: cardiovascular, respiratory and metabolic comorbidities. Pituitary 2017;20(1): 46–62.
8. Ritvonen E, Löyttyniemi E, Jaatinen P, et al. Mortality in acromegaly: a 20-year follow-up study. Endocr Relat Cancer 2016;23(6):469–80.
9. Mercado M, Gonzalez B, Vargas G, et al. Successful mortality reduction and control of comorbidities in patients with acromegaly followed at a highly specialized multidisciplinary clinic. J Clin Endocrinol Metab 2014;99(12):4438–46.
10. Arcopinto M, Bobbio E, Bossone E, et al. The GH/IGF-1 axis in chronic heart failure. Endocrine 2015; 48(1):25–35.
11. Delafontaine P. Insulin like growth factor I and its binding proteins in the cardiovascular system. Cardiovasc Res 1995;30:825–34.
12. D'Ercole AJ, Stiles AD, Underwood LE. Tissue concentrations of somatomedin C: further evidence for multiple sites of synthesis and paracrine or autocrine mechanisms of action. Proc Natl Acad Sci U S A 1984;81:935–9.
13. Ito H, Hiroe M, Hirata Y, et al. Insulin-like growth factor-I induces hypertrophy with enhanced expression of muscle specific genes in cultured rat cardiomyocytes. Circulation 1993;87:1715–21.
14. DeBosch B, Treskov I, Lupu TS, et al. Akt1 is required for physiological cardiac growth. Circulation 2006;113:2097–104.
15. Chen DB, Wang L, Wang PH. Insulin-like growth factor I retards apoptotic signaling induced by ethanol in cardiomyocytes. Life Sci 2000;67:1683–93.
16. Cittadini A, Ishiguro Y, Stroëmer H, et al. Insulin like growth factor-1 but not growth hormone augments mammalian myocardial contractility by sensitizing the myofilament to Ca2þ through a wortmannin-sensitive pathway: studies in rat and ferret isolated muscles. Circ Res 1998;83:50–9.
17. Standley PR, Zhang F, Zayas RM, et al. IGF-I regulation of Na(þ)-K(þ)-ATPase in rat arterial smooth muscle. Am J Physiol 1997;273:E113–21.
18. Anker SD, Al-Nasser FO. Chronic heart failure as a metabolic disorder. Heart Fail Monit 2000;1(2):42–9.
19. Le Corvoisier P, Hittinger L, Chanson P, et al. Cardiac effects of growth hormone treatment in chronic

heart failure: a metaanalysis. J Clin Endocrinol Metab 2007;92:180–5.

20. Saccà L. Growth hormone: a newcomer in cardiovascular medicine. Cardiovasc Res 1997;36:3–9.

21. Niebauer J, Pflaum CD, Clark AL, et al. Deficient insulin-like growth factor I in chronic heart failure predicts altered body composition, anabolic deficiency, cytokine and neurohormonal activation. J Am Coll Cardiol 1998;32:393–7.

22. Cittadini A, Saldamarco L, Marra AM, et al. Growth hormone deficiency in patients with chronic heart failure and beneficial effects of its correction. J Clin Endocrinol Metab 2009;94(9):3329–36.

23. Arcopinto M, Salzano A, Giallauria F, et al, T.O.S.CA. (Trattamento Ormonale Scompenso CArdiaco) Investigators. Growth hormone deficiency is associated with worse cardiac function, physical performance, and outcome in chronic heart failure: insights from the T.O.S.CA. GHD Study. PLoS One 2017;12(1):e0170058.

24. Broglio F, Benso A, Gottero C, et al. Patients with dilated cardiomyopathy show reduction of the somatotroph responsiveness to GHRH both alone and combined with arginine. Eur J Endocrinol 2000; 142(2):157–63.

25. Saccà L, Napoli R, Cittadini A, et al. Growth hormone, acromegaly, and heart failure: an intricate triangulation. Clin Endocrinol (Oxf) 2003;59(6): 660–71.

26. Petersen JW, Felker GM. Inflammatory biomarkers in heart failure. Congest Heart Fail 2006;12:324–8.

27. Al-Obaidi MK, Hon JK, Stubbs PJ, et al. Plasma insulin-like growth factor-1 elevated in mild-to-moderate but not severe heart failure. Am Heart J 2001;142:10.

28. Anker SD, Volterrani M, Pflaum CD, et al. Acquired growth hormone resistance in patients with chronic heart failure: implications for therapy with growth hormone. J Am Coll Cardiol 2001;38: 443–52.

29. Acevedo M, Corbalán R, Chamorro G, et al. Administration of growth hormone to patients with advanced cardiac heart failure: effects upon left ventricular function, exercise capacity, and neurohormonal status. Int J Cardiol 2003;87:185–91.

30. Adamopoulos S, Parissis JT, Paraskevaidis I, et al. Effects of growth hormone on circulating cytokine network, and left ventricular contractile performance and geometry in patients with idiopathic dilated cardiomyopathy. Eur Heart J 2003;24:2186–96.

31. Cittadini A, Ines Comi L, Longobardi S, et al. A preliminary randomized study of growth hormone administration in Becker and Duchenne muscular dystrophies. Eur Heart J 2003;24:664–72.

32. Fazio S, Sabatini D, Capaldo B, et al. A preliminary study of growth hormone in the treatment of dilated cardiomyopathy. N Engl J Med 1996;28:809–14.

33. Frustaci A, Gentiloni N, Russo MA, et al. Growth hormone in the treatment of dilated cardiomyopathy. N Engl J Med 1996;29:672–3.

34. Isgaard J, Bergh CH, Caidahl K, et al. A placebo-controlled study of growth hormone in patients with congestive heart failure. Eur Heart J 1998;19:1704–11.

35. Napoli R, Guardasole V, Matarazzo M, et al. Growth hormone corrects vascular dysfunction in patients with chronic heart failure. J Am Coll Cardiol 2002; 2:90–5.

36. Perrot A, Ranke MB, Dietz R, et al. Growth hormone treatment in dilated cardiomyopathy. J Card Surg 2001;16:127–31.

37. Osterziel KJ, Strohm O, Schuler J, et al. Randomised, double-blind, placebo-controlled trial of human recombinant growth hormone in patients with chronic heart failure due to dilated cardiomyopathy. Lancet 1998;25:1233–7.

38. Petrossians P, Daly AF, Natchev E, et al. Acromegaly at diagnosis in 3173 patients from the Liège Acromegaly Survey (LAS) Database. Endocr Relat Cancer 2017;24(10):505–18.

39. Lombardi G, Di Somma C, Grasso LF, et al. The cardiovascular system in growth hormone excess and growth hormone deficiency. J Endocrinol Invest 2012;35(11):1021–9.

40. Clayton RN. Cardiovascular function in acromegaly. Endocr Rev 2003;24:272–4.

41. Thuesen L, Christensen SE, Weeke J, et al. A hyperkinetic heart in uncomplicated active acromegaly. Explanation of hypertension in acromegalic patients? Acta Med Scand 1988;223:337–43.

42. Castellano G, Affuso F, Conza PD, et al. The GH/IGF-1 axis and heart failure. Curr Cardiol Rev 2009;5(3): 203–15.

43. Brüel A, Christoffersen TE, Nyengaard JR. Growth hormone increases the proliferation of existing cardiac myocytes and the total number of cardiac myocytes in the rat heart. Cardiovasc Res 2007;76(3): 400–8.

44. Hejtmancik MR, Bradfield JY Jr, Herrman GR, et al. Acromegaly and the heart: a clinical and pathologic study. Ann Intern Med 1951;34:1445.

45. Lie JT, Grossman SJ. Pathology of the heart in acromegaly: anatomic findings in 27 autopsied patients. Am Heart J 1980;100:41.

46. Bogazzi F, Lombardi M, Strata E, et al. High prevalence of cardiac hypertrophy without detectable signs of fibrosis in patients with untreated active acromegaly: an in vivo study using magnetic resonance imaging. Clin Endocrinol (Oxf) 2008;68(3): 361–8.

47. dos Santos Silva CM, Gottlieb I, Volschan I, et al. Low frequency of cardiomyopathy using cardiac magnetic resonance imaging in an acromegaly contemporary cohort. J Clin Endocrinol Metab 2015;100(12):4447–55.

48. Colao A, Baldelli R, Marzullo P, et al. Systemic hypertension and impaired glucose tolerance are independently correlated to the severity of the acromegalic cardiomyopathy. J Clin Endocrinol Metab 2000;85:193–9.

49. Bogazzi F, Di Bello V, Palagi C, et al. Improvement of intrinsic myocardial contractility and cardiac fibrosis degree in acromegalic patients treated with somatostatin analogues: a prospective study. Clin Endocrinol (Oxf) 2005;62:590–6.

50. Colao A, Pivonello R, Grasso LF, et al. Determinants of cardiac disease in newly diagnosed patients with acromegaly: results of a 10 year survey study. Eur J Endocrinol 2011;165:713–21.

51. Annamalai AK, Webb A, Kandasamy N, et al. A comprehensive study of clinical, biochemical, radiological, vascular, cardiac, and sleep parameters in an unselected cohort of patients with acromegaly undergoing presurgical somatostatin receptor ligand therapy. J Clin Endocrinol Metab 2013;98:1040–50.

52. Akdeniz BG, Gedik A, Turan O, et al. Evaluation of left ventricular diastolic function according to new criteria and determinants in acromegaly. Int Heart J 2012;53:299–305.

53. Nascimento GC, de Oliveira MT, Carvalho VC, et al. Acromegalic cardiomyopathy in an extensively admixed population: is there a role for GH/IGF-I axis? Clin Endocrinol (Oxf) 2013;78:94–101.

54. Bogazzi F, Lombardi M, Strata E, et al. Effects of somatostatin analogues on acromegalic cardiomyopathy: results from a prospective study using cardiac magnetic resonance. J Endocrinol Invest 2010;33: 103–8.

55. Andreassen M, Faber J, Kjær A, et al. Cardiac effects of 3 months treatment of acromegaly evaluated by magnetic resonance imaging and B-type natriuretic peptides. Pituitary 2010;13:329–36.

56. Maione L, Brue T, Beckers A, et al. Changes in the management and comorbidities of acromegaly over three decades: the French Acromegaly Registry. Eur J Endocrinol 2017;176:645–55.

57. Bihan H, Espinosa C, Valdes-Socin H, et al. Long-term outcome of patients with acromegaly and congestive heart failure. J Clin Endocrinol Metab 2004;89:5308–13.

58. Volschan ICM, Kasuki L, Silva CMS, et al. Two-dimensional speckle tracking echocardiography demonstrates no effect of active acromegaly on left ventricular strain. Pituitary 2017;20:349–57.

59. Di Bello V, Bogazzi F, Di Cori A, et al. Myocardial systolic strain abnormalities in patients with acromegaly: a prospective color Doppler imaging study. J Endocrinol Invest 2006;29:544–50.

60. Geyer H, Caracciolo G, Abe H, et al. Assessment of myocardial mechanics using speckle tracking echocardiography: fundamentals and clinical applications. J Am Soc Echocardiogr 2010;23: 351–69 [quiz: 453–5].

61. Amundsen BH, Helle-Valle T, Edvardsen T, et al. Noninvasive myocardial strain measurement by speckle tracking echocardiography: validation against sonomicrometry and tagged magnetic resonance imaging. J Am Coll Cardiol 2006;47:789–93.

62. Dal J, Feldt-Rasmussen U, Andersen M, et al. Acromegaly incidence, prevalence, complications and long-term prognosis: a nationwide cohort study. Eur J Endocrinol 2016;175(3):181–90.

63. Bogazzi F, Battolla L, Spinelli C, et al. Risk factors for development of coronary heart disease in patients with acromegaly: a five-year prospective study. J Clin Endocrinol Metab 2007;92:4271–7.

64. Akutsu H, Kreutzer J, Wasmeier G, et al. Acromegaly per se does not increase the risk for coronary artery disease. Eur J Endocrinol 2010;162:879–86.

65. Otsuki M, Kasayama S, Yamamoto H, et al. Characterization of premature atherosclerosis of carotid arteries in acromegalic patients. Clin Endocrinol (Oxf) 2001;54:791–6.

66. Boero L, Manavela M, Gómez Rosso L, et al. Alterations in biomarkers of cardiovascular disease (CVD) in active acromegaly. Clin Endocrinol (Oxf) 2009;70:88–95.

67. Corrado E, Rizzo M, Coppola G, et al. An update on the role of markers of inflammation in atherosclerosis. J Atheroscler Thromb 2010;17:1–11.

68. Verhelst J, Velkeniers B, Maiter D, et al. Active acromegaly is associated with decreased hs-CRP and NT-proBNP serum levels: insights from the Belgian registry of acromegaly. Eur J Endocrinol 2013; 168(2):177–84.

69. Sesmilo G, Fairfield WP, Katznelson L, et al. Cardiovascular risk factors in acromegaly before and after normalization of serum IGF-I levels with the GH antagonist pegvisomant. J Clin Endocrinol Metab 2002;87:1692–9.

70. Andreassen M, Faber J, Vestergaard H, et al. N-terminal pro-B-type natriuretic peptide in patients with growth hormone disturbances. Clin Endocrinol (Oxf) 2007;66:619–25.

71. Delaroudis SP, Efstathiadou ZA, Koukoulis GN, et al. Amelioration of cardiovascular risk factors with partial biochemical control of acromegaly. Clin Endocrinol (Oxf) 2008;69:279–84.

72. Kałuzny M, Bolanowski M, Daroszewski J, et al. The role of fibrinogen and CRP in cardiovascular risk in patients with acromegaly. Endokrynol Pol 2010;61: 83–8.

73. Potter BJ, Beauregard C, Serri O. Serum markers of cardiovascular risk in patients with acromegaly before and after six months of treatment with octreotide LAR. Pituitary 2008;11:49–53.

74. Ito M, Kodama M, Tsumanuma I, et al. Relationship between insulin-like growth factor-I and brain

natriuretic peptide in patients with acromegaly after surgery. Circ J 2007;71:1955–7.

75. Arikan S, Bahceci M, Tuzcu A, et al. N-terminal pro-brai natriuretic peptide in newly diagnosed acromegaly. J Endocrinol Invest 2010;33:571–5.

76. Katznelson L, Laws ER Jr, Melmed S, et al, Endocrine Society. Acromegaly: an Endocrine Society clinical practice guideline. J Clin Endocrinol Metab 2014;99:3933–51.

77. Melmed S, Bronstein MD, Chanson P, et al. A consensus statement on acromegaly therapeutic outcomes. Nat Rev Endocrinol 2018;14(9):552–61.

78. Melmed S. New therapeutic agents for acromegaly. Nat Rev Endocrinol 2016;12(2):90–8.

79. Kasuki L, Wildemberg LE, Gadelha MR. Management of endocrine disease: personalized medicine in the treatment of acromegaly. Eur J Endocrinol 2018;178(3):R89–100.

80. Colao A, Vandeva S, Pivonello R, et al. Could different treatment approaches in acromegaly influence life expectancy? A comparative study between Bulgaria and Campania (Italy). Eur J Endocrinol 2014;171:263–73.

81. Colao A, Marzullo P, Cuocolo A, et al. Reversal of acromegalic cardiomyopathy in young but not in middle-aged patients after 12 months of treatment with the depot long acting somatostatin analogue octreotide. Clin Endocrinol (Oxf) 2003;58:169–76.

82. Colao A, Auriemma RS, Galdiero M, et al. Effects of initial therapy for five years with somatostatin analogs for acromegaly on growth hormone and insulin-like growth factor-I levels, tumor shrinkage and cardiovascular disease: a prospective study. J Clin Endocrinol Metab 2009;94(10):3746–56.

83. Colao A, Marzullo P, Ferone D, et al. Cardiovascular effects of depot long-acting somatostatin analog Sandostatin LAR in acromegaly. J Clin Endocrinol Metab 2000;86:3132–40.

84. Giustina A, Casanueva FF, Cavagnini F, et al. Diagnosis and treatment of acromegaly complications. J Endocrinol Invest 2003;26:1242–7.

85. Colao A, Cuocolo A, Marzullo P, et al. Effects of one-year treatment with octreotide on cardiac performance in patients with acromegaly. J Clin Endocrinol Metab 1999;84:17–23.

86. Colao A, Pivonello R, Galderisi M, et al. Impact of treating acromegaly first with surgery or somatostatin analogs on cardiomyopathy. J Clin Endocrinol Metab 2008;93(7):2639–46.

87. Pivonello R, Galderisi M, Auriemma RS, et al. Treatment with growth hormone receptor antagonist in acromegaly: effect on cardiac structure and performance. J Clin Encocrinol Metab 2007;92(2):476–82.

88. Auriemma RS, Grasso LF, Galdiero M, et al. Effects of long-term combined treatment with somatostatin analogues and pegvisomant on cardiac structure and performance in acromegaly. Endocrine 2017; 55(3):872–84.

89. Rajasoorya C, Holdaway IM, Wrightson P, et al. Determinants of clinical outcome and survival in acromegaly. Clin Endocrinol (Oxf) 1994;41:95–102.

β-Adrenergic Receptor Signaling and Heart Failure: From Bench to Bedside

Leonardo Bencivenga, MD[a], Daniela Liccardo, PhD[a],
Carmen Napolitano, MD[a], Lucia Visaggi, MD[a],
Giuseppe Rengo, MD, PhD[a,b], Dario Leosco, MD, PhD[a],*

KEYWORDS

- β-Adrenergic receptors • Heart failure • G-protein-coupled receptors • Therapies • GRK
- β-Arrestin

KEY POINTS

- Increased sympathetic nervous system activity is responsible for β-adrenergic receptor downregulation and desensitization observed in heart failure.
- β-Adrenergic receptor dysfunction plays a crucial role in heart failure pathogenesis, participating in the onset and progression of this syndrome.
- Reactivation of β-adrenergic receptor signaling in heart failure is therapeutic.

HEART FAILURE

Heart failure (HF) is a leading cause of morbidity and mortality worldwide.[1] Its incidence and prevalence increase with age, approaching 10% of the population aged 70 years and older.[1] HF represents the end stage of several cardiovascular diseases (CVDs), such as myocardial infarction, dilated cardiomyopathy, and valvular diseases.[1] The failing heart is not able to ensure adequate perfusion to the rest of the body (systolic dysfunction) and/or to have normal left ventricular (LV) filling, with consequent increased diastolic LV stiffness (diastolic dysfunction).[2] Current guidelines recognize 3 forms of HF based on LV ejection fraction (LVEF): HF with reduced LVEF (ie, less than 40%), HF with preserved LVEF (ie, more than or equal to 50%), and mid-range HF (ie, LVEF between 40% and 49%).[1] The reduction of cardiac output with consequent hypoperfusion of the kidneys and fluid and salt retention are responsible for the main signs and symptoms observed in patients with HF, such as dyspnea, reduced exercise tolerance, increased jugular venous pressure, and ankle swelling.[1] The hyperactivation of neurohormonal systems (adrenergic nervous system [ANS] and renin-angiotensin-aldosterone system) plays a pivotal role in HF pathogenesis.[2] Indeed, β-blockers, angiotensin-converting enzyme inhibitors/sartans, and mineralocorticoid receptor antagonists represent solid pillars of the HF therapeutic armamentarium, because all these drugs have been shown to reduce morbidity and mortality in patients with HF.[1] In particular, the hyperactivation of the sympathetic nervous system (SNS), as shown by increased circulating norepinephrine (NE) levels, initially represents a compensatory mechanism to support cardiac output, but in the long term becomes detrimental, causing or facilitating

Disclosure Statement: The authors have nothing to disclose.
[a] Department of Translational Medical Sciences, Division of Geriatrics, Federico II University, Via Sergio Pansini, 5, Naples 80131, Italy; [b] Istituti Clinici Scientifici Maugeri SpA Società Benefit (ICS Maugeri SpA SB), Telese Terme, Italy
* Corresponding author. Via S. Pansini n. 5, Building 2, 3rd floor, Napoli 80131, Italy.
E-mail address: dleosco@unina.it

Heart Failure Clin 15 (2019) 409–419
https://doi.org/10.1016/j.hfc.2019.02.009

maladaptive ventricular remodeling (increased myocardial fibrosis and apoptosis), reduced exercise tolerance, β-adrenergic receptor (βAR) signaling abnormalities, and increased risk of fatal arrhythmias.[2] Thus, the success of β-blocker therapy lies in its ability to increase survival in patients with HF by blocking the noxious effects of increased catecholamine on the cardiovascular system.[2]

Despite improvements in the management and treatment, mortality rate in patients with HF remains high, approaching 50% at 5 years in symptomatic patients.[1] Thus, deeper knowledge of the mechanisms facilitating HF onset and progression is urgently needed to identify novel therapeutic targets and treatments. This review summarizes the most recent evidence regarding the role of SNS hyperactivity and consequent βAR dysfunction in HF, describing both evidence derived from basic science (bench), and results that have been or will soon be translated to the management and/or treatment of patients with AF (bedside).

β-ADRENERGIC RECEPTOR SIGNALING IN HEART FAILURE

The myocardium is abundantly innervated by adrenergic fibers, involved in compensatory mechanisms including heart-rate acceleration, increased cardiac contractility, accelerated cardiac relaxation, decreased venous capacitance, and constriction of resistance and cutaneous vessels, aiming to ameliorate the performance of the decompensated heart.

SNS activation during HF is characterized by an increase in catecholamine release, NE, and epinephrine (EPI), derived from cardiac sympathetic nerve endings and the adrenal medulla.[3,4] Sympathetic fibers exclusively release NE directly in the cardiac muscle while the chromaffin cells of the adrenal medulla mainly synthesize and release EPI into the blood.[3] Catecholamines mediate their effects through binding to specific adrenergic receptors (ARs), which belong to the superfamily of G-protein–coupled receptors (GPCRs), characterized by a 7-transmembrane domain structure.[3] ARs are divided into 3 types and 9 subtypes: 3 α1AR subtypes (α1A, α1B, α1D), 3 α2AR subtypes (α2A, α2B, α2C), and 3 βAR receptors (β1, β2, β3).[5] Of note, the human heart contains all the 3 types of βARs.[6] β1AR is the predominant subtype in normal hearts, representing 75% to 80% of total βAR density, followed by β2AR (15%–18%) and β3ARs (2%–3%).[7] β1AR and β2AR activation leads to increased cardiac contractility (positive inotropic effect), increased heart rate (positive chronotropic effect), increased rate of relaxation (lusitropic effect), and enhanced impulse conduction through the atrioventricular node (positive dromotropic effect).[8] β3ARs seem to counterbalance cardiac adrenergic overstimulation through a negative inotropic effect, involving the nitric oxide synthase pathway,[9] although the specific function of this AR subtype largely remains unknown. Catecholamine-induced activation of βARs induces the dissociation of guanosine triphosphate (GTP) for guanosine diphosphate (GDP) on the G_α subunit of heterotrimeric G proteins, thus resulting in the dissociation of the heterotrimer into active G_α and free $G_{\beta\gamma}$ subunits, which can transduce intracellular signals.[10] In brief, the signaling cascade after catecholamine-dependent stimulation of cardiomyocyte β1ARs and β2ARs involves the activation of G_s proteins (stimulatory G proteins) which, in turn, stimulate the effector adenylate cyclase (AC) with consequent conversion of adenosine triphosphate (ATP) in cyclic adenosine monophosphate (cAMP), which binds to cAMP-dependent protein kinase (PKA).[10] The increase of free intracellular calcium concentration induced by PKA stimulation promotes cardiac muscle contraction through phosphorylation of different target substrates.[11] The main targets of PKA phosphorylation are: (1) the L-type calcium channels located in the cell membrane and ryanodine receptors located in the sarcoplasmic reticulum both leading to an increase of calcium into the cytoplasm; (2) phospholamban, a negative modulator of sarcoplasmic/endoplasmic reticulum Ca^{2+}-ATPase (SERCA), whose phosphorylation by PKA accelerates Ca^{2+} reuptake by the sarcoplasmic reticulum; and (3) phospholemman whose phosphorylation leads to stimulation of the sodium pump, thus accelerating cardiac muscle repolarization and relaxation.[11,12] PKA can also contribute to βAR uncoupling and desensitization through direct receptor phosphorylation.[13]

With respect to β1ARs, β2AR activation by catecholamines also leads to their coupling to the AC inhibitory G protein (G_i) through the phosphorylation mediated by PKA.[13] This different signaling cascade probably explains why β2AR exerts an antiapoptotic effect in the heart whereas β1AR activation enhances cardiomyocytes apoptosis.[14–17] Furthermore, differences between signaling properties of β1AR and β2AR display important pathophysiologic implications in HF.[18] Indeed, β1ARs are selectively downregulated in HF, as opposed to β2ARs.[19,20] Nevertheless, β1ARs and β2ARs are both functionally uncoupled and desensitized in the failing heart.[2,18–20]

β-ADRENERGIC RECEPTOR POLYMORPHISMS

HF is often associated with genetic βAR polymorphisms also affecting individual responses to β-blocker therapies.[2,21] The most studied gene polymorphism is the Arg389-Gly β1AR, which is associated with enhanced activity of AC/PKA and consequent increase in cardiac contractility.[21] Another β1AR polymorphism is the Ser49Gly, commonly associated with a greater receptor downregulation than the one observed in the Ser49 variant.[22] The Ser49Gly β1AR gene polymorphism is associated with lower prevalence of ventricular arrhythmias and better response to β-blocker therapy.[22–24] The β2AR polymorphisms Gly16Arg and Gln27Glu are involved in receptor downregulation, while a third variation, Thr164Ile, is associated with impaired receptor–G-protein coupling and signal transduction to AC.[24]

G-PROTEIN–COUPLED RECEPTOR KINASES IN HEART FAILURE PATHOPHYSIOLOGY: A NOVEL THERAPEUTIC TARGET

G-Protein–Coupled Receptor Kinase Superfamily

βARs undergo agonist-promoted desensitization and downregulation, aiming to protect the receptors from catecholamine bombardment that is a salient characteristic of HF.[25,26] The molecular mechanisms leading to βAR dysregulation involve receptor phosphorylation by a family of kinases, called G-protein–coupled receptor kinases (GRKs), and binding of β-arrestins to the GRK-phosphorylated receptor. The β-arrestins then uncouple the receptor from G proteins and block the signal transduction to AC.[25,26]

There are 3 groups of GRKs: rhodopsine kinases (GRK1 and GRK7), βAR kinases (GRK2 and GRK3), and GRK4 subfamily (GRK4, GRK5, and GRK6).[27,28]

The GRK structure is based on 3 domains: the amino terminal (N terminal) responsible for receptor binding, a catalytic domain, and the carboxyl terminal (C-terminal) domain interacting with membrane phospholipids.[28] The latter domain is different among the GRK subfamilies and involves several intracellular interactions. The GRK2 C-terminal domain interacts with clathrin that induces βAR internalization, whereas GRK5 C-terminal domain binds membrane phospholipids through electrostatic interactions.[28,29] GRK2 and GRK5 are highly expressed in human heart and may be recognized in almost all cardiac cells, whereas GRK3 has only been detected in cardiac myocytes.[30,31]

In chronic HF and other chronic conditions of ANS hyperactivity, GRK2 is upregulated inside the cardiomyocytes, thus leading to reduction in cardiac βAR density and responsiveness, resulting in cardiac inotropic reserve reduction.[32,33] Interestingly it has been observed that GRK2 upregulation is also evident in peripheral lymphocytes and parallels the increased levels of this kinase in the heart.[34–37] Although GRK2 overexpression possibly represents a protective mechanism against increased catecholamine stimulation, several studies have demonstrated that GRK2 upregulation is noxious for the heart inducing the functional uncoupling of βARs, thus critically affecting βAR-dependent cardiac contractility and function.[38] Experimental studies indicate that overexpression of GRK2 in cardiomyocytes to the same level of upregulation found in human HF (ie, 3- to 4-fold) dramatically blunts βAR signaling and contractile reserve, showing GRK2 to be the main culprit for the functional desensitization of cardiac βARs in HF.[39] Summarizing, increased ANS activity in chronic HF causes enhanced GRK2-mediated cardiac β1-and β2AR desensitization and β1AR downregulation, which lead to the progressive loss of the adrenergic and inotropic reserves of the heart.[40]

Interestingly the increase of GRK2 expression in heart and blood represents an early biomarker for HF diagnosis[41] and prognosis.[34] Moreover, GRK2 is also involved in the βAR-mediated cardiac insulin resistance: previous studies have demonstrated that myocardial β2AR overstimulation and GRK2 upregulation are associated with insulin resistance in the heart.[42]

GRK3 and GRK5 are also involved in the pathogenesis of HF.[43] GRK5 expression is increased in dilated cardiomyopathy and animal and human models of volume-overloaded left ventricle, and cardiac-specific deletion of this kinase induces cardioprotective effects in these cardiac pathologic conditions.[43,44] This evidence implies that regulation of GRK5 in the failing heart may represent an important therapeutic target for HF. On the other hand, GRK3, which belongs to the same subfamily of GRK2, is involved in desensitization of α1AR rather than βAR.

G-Protein–Coupled Receptor Kinase Polymorphisms

GRK5 has an important polymorphism (Leu41Gln), with leucine at position 41 substituted for glutamine, which is largely represented in African Americans.[45,46] This genetic polymorphism leads to a gain of function of the GRK that enhances βAR desensitization and decreases the activity of βAR signaling in a similar manner to that induced by β-blockers. It has been reported that the GRK5-Leu41 polymorphism promotes cardioprotective effects through catecholamines in experimentally induced cardiomyopathies.[45] On the other hand, it has been recently reported that the GRK5 Leu 41 polymorphism is significantly more frequent in Takotsubo patients than in controls (21% versus 6%).[46,47] These data suggest that GRK5 Leu 41 polymorphism is predisposed to cardiac dysfunction caused by sudden and recurring adrenergic stimulation.[46,47] This assertion is in contrast with the aforementioned results demonstrating protection of Leu 41 GRK5 transgenic mice against catecholaminergic cardiomyopathy.[45]

Nevertheless, although referring to a small population, Liggett and colleagues[45] have reported that patients with HF with GRK5-Leu41 show a longer transplant-free survival, thus suggesting GRK5 to constitute a potential target for the treatment of HF.

Therapeutic Approaches of G-Protein–Coupled Receptor Kinases for the Treatment of heart failure

It is known that β-blocker therapy improves the quality of life of patients with HF, limits HF progression, and dramatically improves prognosis for this syndrome. Nevertheless, this class of drugs shows only modest effect in improving contractile function in animal models and humans. A promising therapeutic strategy could be the modulation of GRK expression in the heart to improve the cardiomyocyte response to adrenergic stimulation.[39,48]

In animal models, gene therapy induced overexpression of βARKct, a GRK2 inhibitor, and delayed the progression of functional and biochemical modifications of the βAR signaling associated with HF.[49–51] βARKct is a polypeptide of 194 amino acids with a Gβγ binding domain of GRK2.[51] It competes with the endogenous GRK2 and attenuates GRK2 membrane translocation and activation, thus reducing the GRK2-mediated βAR desensitization.[51] The overexpression of βARKct leads to delay of cardiac dysfunction by preventing negative cardiac remodeling and hypertrophy and improving cardiac function.[51–53] In animal HF models, previous studies have demonstrated that βARKct gene therapy potentiates the beneficial effects of metoprolol.[54] Unfortunately, nowadays, the large molecular size of βARKct and the need for a viral carrier with heart-specific expression limit the clinical development of a gene therapy strategy for human HF.[51]

Of interest, recent studies have focused on the anti-GRK2 activity of paroxetine, a selective serotonin reuptake inhibitor (SSRI) antidepressant[55]: it occupies the active GRK2 kinase domain in a unique inactive form.[56] Moreover, paroxetine has been found to enhance shortening and contraction of isolated cardiac myocytes and to increase βAR-mediated LV inotropic reserve in vivo.[57] All of these effects are independent from the SSRI activity because an equivalent dose of fluoxetine did not show comparable effects.[58] This finding empowers the hypothesis that the effects of paroxetine are due to GRK2 inhibition. These data demonstrate that paroxetine-mediated inhibition of GRK2 enhances cardiac performance, reverses sympathetic overstimulation, normalizes the myocardial βAR function, and protects the heart after myocardial infarction.

ROLE OF β-ARRESTINS IN HEART FAILURE

Four members constitute the arrestin family in vertebrates: arrestins 1 (visual arrestin) and 4 (cone arrestin) are exclusively expressed in the rods and cones of the eyes, respectively; whereas all mammalian tissues, including the cardiovascular system, express β-arrestin 1 (arrestin 2) and β-arrestin 2 (arrestin 3).[59] All arrestins localize in both nucleus and cytoplasm except arrestin 3, which can only be found in the cytoplasm.[60]

β-Arrestins were initially discovered to be terminators of GPCR signaling, including β-AR signaling. Indeed, β-arrestins are recruited after the GRK-mediated βAR phosphorylation, occurring in response to GPCR activation by agonist. This process leads to βAR internalization into cytosol, and consequent receptor degradation or recycling to the cellular membrane, accounting for β-arrestins as key regulators of GPCR endocytosis and trafficking.[61] Furthermore, β-arrestins have been shown to bind many molecules playing a role in HF progression and to act as scaffold protein and signal transducer linking activated GPCR to several intracellular pathways.[62] As already mentioned, the catecholamine binding to βAR produces the coupling of receptor with heterotrimeric G proteins and the dissociation into activated $G_{\alpha s}$ and $G_{\beta \gamma}$ subunits, resulting in an increase of cAMP levels and consequent activated signal transduction. GRKs phosphorylate activated βARs, leading to recruitment of β-arrestins, which prevent further interaction between receptor and G proteins.[26]

Moreover, β-arrestins play a pivotal role in the internalization of receptors into intracellular compartments, a crucial step in trafficking of the GPCRs that have been desensitized.[63] In more detail, this process is realized through binding of β-arrestin to clathrin by the adaptor protein AP2. The 3,4,5-phosphtidylinositols generated on the plasma membrane by phosphoinositide-3-kinase, activated by GRKs, promote association of AP2 to the β-arrestin-clathrin receptor complex, resulting in receptor endocytosis.[64] After internalization, receptors are directed for degradation or recycling via 2 intracellular pathways, which involve lysosomes and enzymatic elimination for receptors targeted to degradation, whereas receptors sorted to recycling are dephosphorylated in acidified vesicles and then carried back to the cellular membrane.[65]

Importantly, β-arrestins also act as adaptor proteins or effectors to downstream signaling, including JNK, ERK1/2, and Src pathways.[66–68] Finally, β-arrestins show ability to form complexes of multimolecular proteins. Mangmool and colleagues[69] have demonstrated that activated β1ARs produce conformational change in β-arrestin, making it able to determine a stable complex with Ca^{2+}/calmodulin kinase II (CaMKII) and cAMP-dependent guanine-nucleotide exchange factor (Epac). The resulting complex, which is not observed for the β2AR, leads Epac and CaMKII to structural proximity, resulting in CaMKII signaling activation. These processes seem to be involved in the pathogenesis of cardiac hypertrophy and HF.[69]

Cardioprotective Versus Cardiotoxic Effects

Whereas β-arrestin 1 may be considered detrimental under pathologic conditions through β1AR desensitization and via activation of proapoptotic and proinflammatory signaling, β-arrestin 2 generally counteracts cell death signaling.

McCrink and colleagues[70] have shown a restoration of the inotropic reserve by overexpressing β-arrestin 2 in a mouse model of myocardial infarction. Mechanistically these protective effects seem to involve direct binding and activation of sarcoplasmic/endoplasmic reticulum Ca^{2+}-ATPase2a (SERCA2a), which plays a crucial role in the regulation of cardiac contractility. The investigators also demonstrated an increase in SERCA2a SUMO (small ubiquitin-like modifier)-ylation and activity, leading to a reduction in adverse remodeling caused by fibrosis and apoptosis. Another beneficial effect of β-arrestin 2 involves the inflammatory response to myocardial injury. Indeed, β-arrestin 2 delays inflammatory processes as demonstrated by the increase in inflammatory cytokines levels in β-arrestin 2 knockout (KO) mice after myocardial infarction.[71] Moreover, a role for β-arrestin 2 has been described in the inhibition of excessive inflammation and prevention

of myocyte apoptosis.[72] Conversely, a recent report by Wang and colleagues[73] points out the upregulation of β-arrestin 2 to be detrimental in in vivo/in vitro models of cardiac ischemia/reperfusion injury, highlighting the need to better define the mechanisms underlying these conditions.

Investigations regarding the role of β-arrestin 1 in postmyocardial infarction remodeling have been conducted using β-arrestin 1 KO mice, which showed better overall cardiac function, increased survival, and reduced infarct size, apoptosis, and adverse remodeling compared with wild-type mice.

Summarizing, β-arrestin 1 probably constitutes the β-arrestin isoform responsible for βAR desensitization and downregulation, participating in HF pathophysiology, whereas stimulation of β-arrestin 2 seems to promote cell survival and proliferation.[74]

Biased Agonism

A β-arrestin–biased ligand selectively activates β-arrestin signaling pathway, independently from the G-protein signaling, which in turn results in antagonism.[75] Owing to the functional selectivity in the activation of G-protein–independent β-arrestin signaling, a β-arrestin–biased ligand is considered able to exert protective effects on HF progression through the stabilization of βAR in a different inactive conformation.[62]

Long-term administration of β-blockers is known to clinically delay HF progression, resulting in reduction of cardiac remodeling and improvement in LV contractility.[76] The mechanisms underlying the protective effects of β-blocker therapy include the reactivation of β1AR function. Accordingly, the use of this class of drug has been demonstrated to augment βAR function and to diminish GRK2 expression levels.[77] It is well known that, β-blocker family members show several differences regarding βAR isoform selectivity and power of action on αAR, antioxidant, and anti-inflammatory activities. Importantly some β-blockers, including carvedilol, express bias toward β-arrestin–dependent signaling, resulting in epidermal growth factor receptor (EGFR) and ERK1/2 activation, independently of $G_{\alpha s}$ protein activity. Furthermore, β1AR polymorphisms have been associated with β-arrestin 2 cardiomyocyte hegemony in response to carvedilol[78]; moreover, cardiac levels of certain microRNAs, related to cell survival and apoptosis repression, were enhanced by carvedilol in ischemia-reperfusion models.[79,80] Otherwise, a clinical benefit did not emerge in a recent meta-analysis comparing carvedilol and the unbiased agonist metoprolol in patients with HF,[81] once again underlining the need for further studies on dosages or alternative therapeutic approaches.

New therapeutic perspectives are emerging in the research area of allosteric modulators in hopes of discovering molecules able to promote β-arrestin–biased signaling. β2AR-specific pepducins, lipidated peptides in GPCR intracellular loops, have been developed to selectively activate biased signaling through either G_s- or β-arrestin–dependent pathways[82]; a study in human embryonic kidney cells has confirmed their ability to activate the EGFR and ERK1/2 pathways and to also improve cardiomyocyte contractility, regardless of canonic βAR pathway.[83]

INTERACTION BETWEEN β-ADRENERGIC RECEPTORS AND OTHER RECEPTOR SYSTEMS

The term receptor crosstalk was first used in the early 1980s to explain some unexpected behaviors of certain pharmacologic agents, such as GPCR agonists.[84] For instance, in isolated rat hearts, Lochner and coworkers[85] observed that αAR-agonism inhibited βAR activity. Similarly, Lemire and colleagues[86] demonstrated that βAR-mediated activation of AC is impaired in the heart of mice overexpressing the αAR. Thus, the phenomenon of crosstalk has been defined in a more generic way as the ability of a receptor to transactivate other receptor systems and/or determine the activation of multiple cellular signaling pathways.[84] At cardiac level the crosstalk phenomenon has been identified in different cell types, and it seems to involve several receptors (GPCR and non-GPCR) playing a prominent role in the regulation of heart function.[84] Importantly one of the most exhaustively investigated crosstalks is that observed between the β1AR and the angiotensin 2 type 1 receptor (AT1R). In this context, Schwartz and Naff[87] proved that, in rat heart, angiotensin II–mediated AT1R stimulation resulted in protein kinase C activation with consequent decreased β1AR responsiveness. Analogously, in cell cultures Gelband and colleagues[88] observed G_i proteins to stimulate downstream AT1R-inhibited βAR-mediated AC activity. Conversely, in 2003 Barki-Harrington and colleagues[89] demonstrated in cardiomyocytes the presence of a physical interaction between β1AR and AT1R. Indeed, βAR blockade via propranolol was able to inhibit the angiotensin II–mediated contractility. Analogously, these investigators proved that the blockade of the AT1R resulted in the inhibition of the effects on the heart rate induced by βAR stimulation.

Another important relevant mechanism of crosstalk is that observed between the β1AR and the EGFR by Noma and colleagues.[72] More specifically, these investigators have demonstrated that an increase in circulating catecholamine, with consequent β1AR activation, induced the recruitment of β-arrestin proteins and the consequent activation of the kinase c-Src3. Of note, c-Src led to the activation of matrix metalloproteinases that promoted the release of EGF-like heparin binding factor and the subsequent activation of the EGFR.[72] Notably this mechanism appears to be a protective response of cardiomyocytes activated under stress conditions. Therefore, given the great importance of the crosstalk mechanisms in cardiac pathophysiology, during the last 10 years the authors' research group has also focused its interest on studying these pathways to identify novel potential therapeutic targets (**Fig. 1**). In this regard they have demonstrated that βAR hyperstimulation negatively affects insulin receptor signaling in cardiomyocytes, a particularly relevant mechanism because it helps to explain, at least in part, the onset of insulin resistance in postischemic failing myocardium. Of note, the authors have demonstrated that following catecholamine stimulation of cardiomyocytes the kinase GRK2 is upregulated, leading to the inhibition of insulin signaling through direct binding and phosphorylation of the insulin receptor substrate 1.[90] Analogously, Fu and colleagues[91] have observed that the hyperactivation of GRK2, following insulin receptor stimulation, induced the phosphorylation and desensitization of β2AR in cardiomyocytes.

In a recent study the authors also identified, at cardiomyocyte level, the existence of an interaction between the β1AR and the sphingosine 1-phosphate (S1P) type 1 receptor (S1PR1).[92] The S1PR1 mediates in the heart the effects of the bioactive lipid S1P with multiple activities such as the stimulation of endothelial function and the inhibition of cardiomyocyte apoptosis.[93] Interestingly, previous studies have demonstrated that S1PR1, through its coupling with G_i protein, produces a signaling able to block β1AR-mediated AC activation.[94] In line with these data, the authors' group has demonstrated the presence in cardiomyocytes of a direct crosstalk between β1AR and S1PR1, which is finely orchestrated by GRK2. It is noteworthy that such a mechanism seems to play a crucial role in the pathogenesis of postischemic HF.[92] Indeed, the increased SNS activity, and the consequent β1AR hyperactivation, induces an augmented GRK2 expression/activity that reciprocally downregulates both β1AR and S1PR1, with a consequent negative

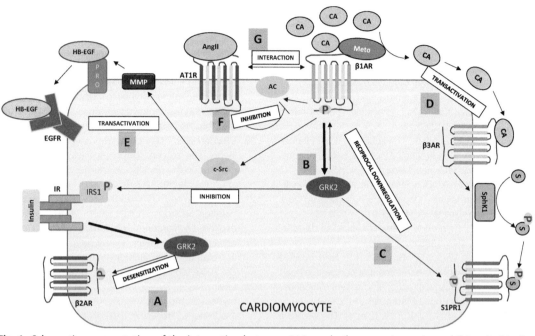

Fig. 1. Schematic representation of the interaction between βARs and other receptor systems. (*A*) Insulin binding to insulin receptor (IR) results in upregulation of GRK2, which in turn desensitizes the β2AR. (*B*) GRK2 is also up-regulated in response to increased catecholamines (CA) and to β1AR hyperstimulation. (*C*) Of note, GRK2 induces the phosphorylation and reciprocal downregulation of both β1AR and S1PR1. (*D*) Metoprolol (Meto) inhibits catecholamine binding to β1AR and transports them to the β3AR (transactivation mechanism). Importantly, the sphingosine kinase 1 (SphK1) is activated downstream of β3AR activation leading to S1P generation and S1PR1 activation. (*E*) In response to catecholamine stimulation of β1AR, there is activation of c-Src and the matrix metalloproteinases (MMP) that in turn leads to the release of heparin-bound epidermal growth factor (HB-EGF) with activation of epidermal growth factor receptor (EGFR). (*F*) Angiotensin II (AngII) stimulation of AT1R inhibits the adenylyl cyclase (AC) activation mediated by β1AR. (*G*) The AT1R and β1AR can physically interact (heterodimerization).

effect on LV function and remodeling. Furthermore, the authors have also shown that selective β1 blockade may prevent dysregulation of the S1PR1 receptor, thus inducing a better response to ischemic damage.[95] In particular, these data demonstrated that β1AR blockade, by metoprolol, transports more catecholamine to the β3AR, thus mediating "transactivation" of this latter βAR subtype.[95] As a consequence of this mechanism, the β3AR induces an increased production and release of S1P through the activation of the sphingosine kinase 1 (the rate-limiting enzyme for S1P production), thus resulting in a better cardiac function and remodeling after myocardial infarction.[93,95]

SUMMARY

SNS hyperactivity and consequent abnormalities in βAR signaling are considered as the major culprits of HF development and progression. Indeed, correction of βAR dysfunction, at receptor level, has been recognized as a valid strategy

against HF (ie, β-blocker therapy). Furthermore, the identification of receptor crosstalk mechanisms between βAR and other GPCRs and non-GPCRs in cardiomyocytes has upset the classical idea that stimulation of a receptor could determine the activation of a single molecular pathway. Therefore, a deeper knowledge of the mechanisms underlying HF-related βAR signaling alterations will allow the development of more specific therapeutic strategies for better management of patients with this prevalent syndrome.

REFERENCES

1. Ponikowski P, Voors AA, Anker SD, et al. 2016 ESC Guidelines for the diagnosis and treatment of acute and chronic heart failure: The Task Force for the diagnosis and treatment of acute and chronic heart failure of the European Society of Cardiology (ESC) developed with the special contribution of the Heart Failure Association (HFA) of the ESC. Eur Heart J 2016;37:2129–200.

2. Lymperopoulos A, Rengo G, Koch WJ. Adrenergic nervous system in heart failure: pathophysiology and therapy. Circ Res 2013;113:739–53.

3. Lymperopoulos A, Rengo G, Koch WJ. Adrenal adrenoceptors in heart failure: fine-tuning cardiac stimulation. Trends Mol Med 2007;13:503–11.

4. Lymperopoulos A. Ischemic emergency? endothelial cells have their own "adrenaline shot" at hand. Hypertension 2012;60:12–4.

5. Bylund DB, Eikenberg DC, Hieble JP, et al. International Union of Pharmacology nomenclature of adrenoreceptors. Pharmacol Rev 1994;46:121–36.

6. Lymperopoulos A, Rengo G, Koch WJ. GRK2 inhibition in heart failure: something old, something new. Curr Pharm Des 2012;18:186–91.

7. Brodde OE. Beta-adrenoceptors in cardiac disease. Pharmacol Ther 1993;60:405–30.

8. Colucci WS, Wright RF, Braunwald E. New positive inotropic agents in the treatment of congestive heart failure. Mechanisms of action and recent clinical developments. N Engl J Med 1986;314:290–9.

9. Gauthier C, Leblais V, Kobzik L, et al. The negative inotropic effect of beta3-adrenoceptor stimulation is mediated by activation of a nitric oxide synthase pathway in human ventricle. J Clin Invest 1998; 102:1377–84.

10. Lohse MJ, Engelhardt S, Eschenhagen T. What is the role of beta-adrenergic signaling in heart failure? Circ Res 2003;93:896–906.

11. Bers DM. Calcium cycling and signaling in cardiac myocytes. Annu Rev Physiol 2008;70:23–49.

12. Despa S, Bossuyt J, Han F, et al. Phospholemman-phosphorylation mediates the beta-adrenergic effects on Na/K pump function in cardiac myocytes. Circ Res 2005;97:252–9.

13. Daaka Y, Luttrell LM, Lefkowitz RJ. Switching of the coupling of the beta2-adrenergic receptor to different G proteins by protein kinase A. Nature 1997;390:88–91.

14. Communal C, Singh K, Sawyer DB, et al. Opposing effects of β1- and β2-adrenergic receptors on cardiac myocyte apoptosis: role of a pertussis toxin-sensitive G protein. Circulation 1999;100:2210–2.

15. Chesley A, Lundberg MS, Asai T, et al. The β2-adrenergic receptor delivers an antiapoptotic signal to cardiac myocytes through Gi-dependent coupling to phosphatidylinositol 3-kinase. Circ Res 2000;87:1172–9.

16. Zhu WZ, Zheng M, Koch WJ, et al. Dual modulation of cell survival and cell death by β2- adrenergic signaling in adult mouse cardiomyocyte. Proc Natl Acad Sci U S A 2001;98:1607–12.

17. Dorn GW II, Tepe NM, Lorenz JN, et al. Low and high level transgenic expression of β2- adrenergic receptors differentially affect cardiac hypertrophy and function in Gaq-overexpressing mice. Proc Natl Acad Sci U S A 1999;96:6400–5.

18. Rockman HA, Koch WJ, Lefkowitz RJ. Seven-trans membrane-spanning receptors and heart function. Nature 2002;415:206–12.

19. Bristow MR, Ginsburg R, Umans V, et al. β1- and β2 adrenergic-receptor subpopulations in nonfailing and failing human ventricular myocardium: coupling of both receptor subtypes to muscle contraction and selective β1-receptor down-regulation in heart failure. Circ Res 1986;59:297–309.

20. Bristow MR, Ginsburg R, Minobe W, et al. Decreased catecholamine sensitivity and β-adrenergic receptor density in failing human hearts. N Engl J Med 1982;307:205–11.

21. Sandilands AJ, O'Shaughnessy KM, Brown MJ. Greater inotropic and cyclic AMP responses evoked by noradrenaline through Arg389 beta1 adrenoceptors versus Gly389 beta1-adrenoceptors in isolated human atrial myocardium. Br J Pharmacol 2003;138:386–92.

22. Levin MC, Marullo S, Muntaner O, et al. The myocardium-protective Gly-49 variant of the beta 1-adrenergic receptor exhibits constitutive activity and increased desensitization and down-regulation. J Biol Chem 2002;277:30429–35.

23. Borjesson M, Magnusson Y, Hjalmarson A, et al. A novel polymorphism in the gene coding for the beta(1)-adrenergic receptor associated with survival in patients with heart failure. Eur Heart J 2000;21 1853–8.

24. Johnson JA, Liggett SB. Cardiovascular pharmacogenomics of adrenergic receptor signaling: clinical implications and future directions. Clin Pharmacol Ther 2011;89:366–78.

25. Reiter E, Lefkowitz RJ. GRKs and beta-arrestins roles in receptor silencing, trafficking and signaling. Trends Endocrinol Metab 2006;17:159–65.

26. Ferguson SS. Evolving concepts in G protein coupled receptor endocytosis: the role in receptor desensitization and signaling. Pharmacol Rev 2001;53:1–24.

27. Penn RB, Pronin AN, Benovic JL. Regulation of G protein-coupled receptor kinases. Trends Cardiovasc Med 2000;10:81–9.

28. Penela P, Ribas C, Mayor F Jr. Mechanisms of regulation of the expression and function of G protein coupled receptor kinases. Cell Signal. 2003;15 973–81.

29. Mangmool S, Haga T, Kobayashi H, et al. Clathrin required for phosphorylation and internalization of β2-adrenergic receptor by G protein-coupled receptor kinase 2 (GRK2). J Biol Chem 2006;281:31940–9.

30. Vinge LE, Oie E, Andersson Y, et al. Myocardial distribution and regulation of GRK and β-arrestin isoforms in congestive heart failure in rats. Am J Physiol Heart Circ Physiol 2001;281:H2490–9.

31. Penela P, Murga C, Ribas C, et al. Mechanisms of regulation of G protein-coupled receptor kinases

(GRKs) and cardiovascular disease. Cardiovasc Res 2006;69:46–56.

32. Rengo G, Lymperopoulos A, Koch WJ. Future G protein-coupled receptor targets for treatment of heart failure. Curr Treat Options Cardiovasc Med 2009;11:328–38.

33. Floras JS. The "unsympathetic" nervous system of heart failure. Circulation 2002;105:1753–5.

34. Rengo G, Pagano G, Filardi PP, et al. Prognostic value of lymphocyte G protein-coupled receptor kinase-2 protein levels in patients with heart failure. Circ Res 2016;118:1116–24.

35. Iaccarino G, Barbato E, Cipolletta E, et al. Elevated myocardial and lymphocyte GRK2 expression and activity in human heart failure. Eur Heart J 2005;26: 1752–8.

36. Femminella GD, Rengo G, Pagano G, et al. β-Adrenergic receptors and G protein-coupled receptor kinase-2 in Alzheimer's disease: a new paradigm for prognosis and therapy? J Alzheimers Dis 2013; 34:341–7.

37. Leosco D, Fortunato F, Rengo G, et al. Lymphocyte G-protein-coupled receptor kinase-2 is upregulated in patients with Alzheimer's disease. Neurosci Lett 2007;415:279–82.

38. Ungerer M, Böhm M, Elce JS, et al. Altered expression of beta-adrenergic receptor kinase and beta 1-adrenergic receptors in the failing human heart. Circulation 1993;87:454–63.

39. Koch WJ, Rockman HA, Samama P, et al. Cardiac function in mice overexpressing the β-adrenergic receptor kinase or a βARK inhibitor. Science 1995;268: 1350–3.

40. Eschenhagen T. Beta-adrenergic signaling in heart failure-adapt or die. Nat Med 2008;14:485–7.

41. Rengo G, Lymperopoulos A, Leosco D, et al. GRK2 as a novel gene therapy target in heart failure. J Mol Cell Cardiol 2011;50:785–92.

42. Mangmool S, Denkaew T, Parichatikanond W, et al. β-Adrenergic receptor and insulin resistance in the heart. Biomol Ther (Seoul) 2017;25:44–56.

43. Dzimiri N, Muiya P, Andres E, et al. Differential functional expression of human myocardial G protein receptor kinases in left ventricular cardiac diseases. Eur J Pharmacol 2004;489:167–77.

44. Gold JI, Gao E, Shang X, et al. Determining the absolute requirement of G-coupled receptor kinase 5 for pathological cardiac hypertrophy: short communication. Circ Res 2012;115:976–85.

45. Liggett SB, Cresci S, Kelly RJ, et al. A GRK5 polymorphism that inhibits β-adrenergic receptor signaling is protective in heart failure. Nat Med 2008;14:510–7.

46. Spinelli L, Trimarco V, Di Marino S, et al. L41q polymorphism of the G protein coupled receptor kinase 5 is associated with left ventricular apical ballooning syndrome. Eur J Heart Fail 2010;12:13–6.

47. Dorn GW 2nd. Adrenergic signaling polymorphisms and their impact on cardiovascular disease. Physiol Rev 2010;90:1013–62.

48. Korzick D, Xiao R, Ziman B, et al. Transgenic manipulation of beta-adrenergic receptor kinase modifies cardiac myocyte contraction to norepinephrine. Am J Physiol 1997;272:H590–6.

49. Rockman HA, Chien KR, Choi DJ, et al. Expression of a β-adrenergic receptor kinase 1 inhibitor prevents the development of myocardial failure in gene-targeted mice. Proc Natl Acad Sci U S A 1998;95:7000–5.

50. Hullmann J, Traynham CJ, Coleman RC, et al. The expanding GRK interactome: implications in cardiovascular disease and potential for therapeutic development. Pharmacol Res 2016;110:52–64.

51. Cannavo A, Komici K, Bencivenga L, et al. GRK2 as a therapeutic target for heart failure. Expert Opin Ther Targets 2018;22:75–83.

52. White DC, Hata JA, Shah AS, et al. Preservation of myocardial β-adrenergic receptor signaling delays the development of heart failure after myocardial infarction. Proc Natl Acad Sci U S A 2000;97: 5428–33.

53. Shah AS, White DC, Emani S, et al. In vivo ventricular gene delivery of a β-adrenergic receptor kinase inhibitor to the failing heart reverses cardiac dysfunction. Circulation 2001;103:1311–6.

54. Harding VB, Jones LR, Lefkowitz RJ, et al. Cardiac βARK1 inhibition prolongs survival and augments β-blocker therapy in a mouse model of severe heart failure. Proc Natl Acad Sci U S A 2001;98:5809–14.

55. Homan KT, Wu E, Wilson MW, et al. Structural and functional analysis of G protein-coupled receptor kinase inhibition by paroxetine and a rationally designed analog. Mol Pharmacol 2014;85: 237–48.

56. Thal DM, Yeow RY, Schoenau C, et al. Molecular, mechanism of selectivity among G protein-coupled receptor kinase 2 inhibitors. Mol Pharmacol 2011; 80:294–303.

57. Thal DM, Homan KT, Chen J, et al. Paroxetine is a direct inhibitor of G protein-coupled receptor kinase 2 and increases myocardial contractility. ACS Chem Biol 2012;7:1830–9.

58. Schumacher SM, Gao E, Zhu W, et al. Paroxetine-mediated GRK2 inhibition reverses and remodeling after myocardial infarction. Sci Transl Med 2015;7: 277ra31.

59. Lefkowitz RJ, Shenoy SK. Transduction of receptor signals by beta-arrestins. Science 2005;308:512–7.

60. Oakley RH, Laporte SA, Holt JA, et al. Differential affinities of visual arrestin, beta arrestin1, and beta arrestin2 for G protein-coupled receptors delineate two major classes of receptors. J Biol Chem 2000; 275:17201–10.

61. Moore CAC, Milano SK, Benovic JL. Regulation of receptor trafficking by GRKs and arrestins. Annu Rev Physiol 2007;69:451–82.

62. Noor N, Patel CB, Rockman HA, et al. A signaling molecule and potential therapeutic target for heart failure. J Mol Cell Cardiol 2011;51:534–41.

63. Sibley DR, Strasser RH, Benovic JL, et al. Phosphorylation/dephosphorylation of the beta-adrenergic receptor regulates its functional coupling to adenylate cyclase and subcellular distribution. Proc Natl Acad Sci U S A 1986;83:9408–12.

64. Lefkowitz R, Ahn S, Lefkowitz RJ, et al. Introduction to special section on β-arrestins. Annu Rev Physiol 2007;69. https://doi.org/10.1146/annurev.ph.69.013107.100021.

65. Tan CM, Brady AE, Nickols HH, et al. Membrane trafficking of G protein-coupled receptors. Annu Rev Pharmacol Toxicol 2004;44:559–609.

66. Luttrell LM, Ferguson SS, Daaka Y, et al. Beta-arrestin-dependent formation of beta2 adrenergic receptor-Src protein kinase complexes. Science 1999;283:655–61.

67. McDonald PH, Chow CW, Miller WE, et al. Beta-arrestin 2: a receptor-regulated MAPK scaffold for the activation of JNK3. Science 2000;290:1574–7.

68. Shenoy SK, Drake MT, Nelson CD, et al. β-Arrestin-dependent, G protein-independent ERK1/2 activation by the β2 adrenergic receptor. J Biol Chem 2006;281:1261–73.

69. Mangmool S, Shukla AK, Rockman HA. β-Arrestin-dependent activation of Ca^{2+}/calmodulin kinase II after β1-adrenergic receptor stimulation. J Cell Biol 2010;189:573–87.

70. McCrink KA, Maning J, Vu A, et al. β-Arrestin2 improves post-myocardial infarction heart failure via sarco(endo)plasmic reticulum Ca^{2+}-ATPase-dependent positive inotropy in cardiomyocytes. Hypertension 2017;70:972–81.

71. Watari K, Nakaya M, Kurose H. Multiple functions of G protein-coupled receptor kinases. J Mol Signal 2014;9(1):1.

72. Noma T, Lemaire A, Naga Prasad SV, et al. β-Arrestin-mediated β1-adrenergic receptor transactivation of the EGFR confers cardioprotection. J Clin Invest 2007;117:2445–58.

73. Wang Y, Jin L, Song Y, et al. β-Arrestin 2 mediates cardiac ischemia-reperfusion injury via inhibiting GPCR-independent cell survival signalling. Cardiovasc Res 2017;113:1615–26.

74. Bathgate-Siryk A, Dabul S, Pandya K, et al. Negative impact of β-arrestin-1 on post-myocardial infarction heart failure via cardiac and adrenal-dependent neurohormonal mechanisms. Hypertension 2014; 63:404–12.

75. Wisler JW, Xiao K, Thomsen AR, et al. Recent developments in biased agonism. Curr Opin Cell Biol 2014;27:18–24.

76. López-Sendón J, Swedberg K, McMurray J, et al. Task Force on Beta-Blockers of the European Society of Cardiology. Expert consensus document on beta-adrenergic receptor blockers. Eur Heart J 2004;25:1341–62.

77. Iaccarino G, Tomhave ED, Lefkowitz RJ, et al. Reciprocal in vivo regulation of myocardial G protein-coupled receptor kinase expression by beta-adrenergic receptor stimulation and blockade. Circulation 1998;98:1783–9.

78. McCrink KA, Brill A, Jafferjee M, et al. β1-adrenoceptor Arg389Gly polymorphism confers differential β-arrestin-binding tropism in cardiac myocytes. Pharmacogenomics 2016;17:1611–20.

79. Bayoumi AS, Park K, Wang Y, et al. A carvedilol-responsive microRNA, miR-125b-5p protects the heart from acute myocardial infarction by repressing pro-apoptotic bak1 and klf13 in cardiomyocytes. J Mol Cell Cardiol 2018;114:72–82.

80. Park K-M, Teoh J-P, Wang Y, et al. Carvedilol-responsive microRNAs, miR-199a-3p and -214 protect cardiomyocytes from simulated ischemia-reperfusion injury. Am J Physiol Heart Circ Physiol 2016;311 H371–83.

81. Briasoulis A, Palla M, Afonso L. Meta-analysis of the effects of carvedilol versus metoprolol on all-cause mortality and hospitalizations in patients with heart failure. Am J Cardiol 2015;115:1111–5.

82. Carr R, Du Y, Quoyer J, et al. Development and characterization of pepducins as Gs-biased allosteric agonists. J Biol Chem 2014;289 35668–84.

83. Carr R, Schilling J, Song J, et al. β-arrestin-biased signaling through the β2-adrenergic receptor promotes cardiomyocyte contraction. Proc Natl Acad Sci U S A 2016;113:E4107–16.

84. Dzimiri N. Receptor crosstalk. Implications for cardiovascular function, disease and therapy. Eur J Biochem 2002;269:4713–30.

85. Lochner A, Tromp E, Mouton R. Signal transduction in myocardial ischaemia and reperfusion. Mol Cell Biochem 1996;160-161:129–36.

86. Lemire I, Allen BG, Rindt H, et al. Cardiac-specific overexpression of alpha1BAR regulates betaAR activity via molecular crosstalk. J Mol Cell Cardiol 1998;30:1827–39.

87. Schwartz DD, Naff BP. Activation of protein kinase C by angiotensin II decreases beta 1-adrenergic receptor responsiveness in the rat heart. J Cardiovasc Pharmacol 1997;29:257–64.

88. Gelband CH, Sumners C, Lu D, et al. Angiotensin receptors and norepinephrine neuromodulation: implications of functional coupling. Regul Pept 1998;73 141–7.

89. Barki-Harrington L, Luttrell LM, Rockman HA. Dual inhibition of beta-adrenergic and angiotensin II receptors by a single antagonist: a functional role for

receptor-receptor interaction in vivo. Circulation 2003;108:1611–8.

90. Ciccarelli M, Chuprun JK, Rengo G, et al. G protein-coupled receptor kinase 2 activity impairs cardiac glucose uptake and promotes insulin resistance after myocardial ischemia. Circulation 2011;123:1953–62.

91. Fu Q, Xu B, Parikh D, et al. Insulin induces IRS2-dependent and GRK2-mediated β2AR internalization to attenuate βAR signaling in cardiomyocytes. Cell Signal 2015;27:707–15.

92. Cannavo A, Rengo G, Liccardo D, et al. β1-adrenergic receptor and sphingosine-1-phosphate receptor 1 (S1PR1) reciprocal downregulation influences cardiac hypertrophic response and progression to heart failure: protective role of S1PR1 cardiac gene therapy. Circulation 2013;128:1612–22.

93. Cannavo A, Liccardo D, Komici K, et al. Sphingosine kinases and sphingosine 1-phosphate receptors: signaling and actions in the cardiovascular system. Front Pharmacol 2017;8:556.

94. Means CK, Miyamoto S, Chun J, et al. S1P1 receptor localization confers selectivity for Gi-mediated cAMP and contractile responses. J Biol Chem 2008;283:11954–63.

95. Cannavo A, Rengo G, Liccardo D, et al. β1-blockade prevents post-ischemic myocardial decompensation via β3AR-dependent protective sphingosine-1 phosphate signaling. J Am Coll Cardiol 2017;70:182–92.

Evaluation of Cardiac Metabolism by Magnetic Resonance Spectroscopy in Heart Failure

Santo Dellegrottaglie, MD, PhD[a,b,*], Alessandra Scatteia, MD[a], Carmine Emanuele Pascale, RT[a], Francesco Renga, MD[c], Pasquale Perrone-Filardi, MD, PhD[c]

KEYWORDS

- Heart failure • Magnetic resonance • Noninvasive imaging • Cardiac metabolism

KEY POINTS

- Although cardiac magnetic resonance spectroscopy (MRS) is currently mostly limited to the research setting, increasing evidence demonstrates its ability to provide important insights into myocardial energetic metabolism in various cardiac disease conditions, including heart failure.
- In patients with heart failure, ^{1}H-MRS mainly allows investigation of the contribution of myocardial lipid accumulation and lipotoxicity to the development and clinical course of the disease.
- ^{31}P-MRS can provide direct information of myocardial metabolic health, principally through the assessment of the adenosine triphosphate to phosphocreatine ratio (PCr/ATP ratio), which is typically reduced in the failing heart and correlates with cardiac functional status.
- Recent technical and methodological developments with MRS have the potential to strengthen the capacity to investigate cardiac pathophysiology, finally enabling application of cardiac MRS in clinical practice for initial characterization and successive monitoring of patients with heart failure.

INTRODUCTION

Heart failure (HF) is a major and growing health problem worldwide, associated with relevant morbidity, mortality, and economic costs.[1] Multiple potential causes can lead to HF development, resulting in the heterogeneous phenotypes clinically observed. Unfortunately, the complex pathophysiologic mechanisms involved in the development of HF are only partially understood and this may be one of the reason justifying the limited long-term efficacy frequently encountered with available treatment strategies.[2]

MRI is a widely diffuse diagnostic modality that can produce detailed anatomic images throughout the human body, based on the physical phenomenon called nuclear magnetic resonance. Magnetic resonance spectroscopy (MRS) is a clinically less-diffuse application of nuclear magnetic resonance and provides a noninvasive method for characterizing chemistry and cellular features in vivo. It allows the detection of relatively small molecules in intracellular and extracellular spaces. The obtained information about different tissues offers the possibility to monitor metabolic changes

Disclosure: The authors have nothing to disclose.
[a] Division of Cardiology, Ospedale Accreditato Villa dei Fiori, Acerra, Naples, Italy; [b] Zena and Michael A. Wiener Cardiovascular Institute/Marie-Josee and Henry R. Kravis Center for Cardiovascular Health, Icahn School of Medicine at Mount Sinai, New York, NY, USA; [c] Department of Advanced Biomedical Sciences, University of Naples Federico II, Naples, Italy
* Corresponding author. Cardiovascular MRI Laboratory, Division of Cardiology, Ospedale Accreditato Villa dei Fiori, Corso Italia, 157 - Acerra, Naples 81100, Italy.
E-mail address: sandel74@hotmail.com

caused by disease and to assess effects of treatment.[3]

Nuclear magnetic resonance is based on the property of certain atoms to produce a net and measurable magnetic moment. In particular, this can be observed with nuclei with an odd number of protons, such as phosphorus 31 (^{31}P), carbon 13 (^{13}C), sodium 23 (^{23}Na), rubidium 87 (^{87}Rb), and, most importantly, hydrogen 1 (^{1}H). Compounds containing these nuclei are involved in the major metabolic processes typically observed in the viable myocardium, including high-energy phosphate metabolism, Krebs cycle, and fatty acid metabolism.[4] MRS was applied to study cardiac metabolism for the first time about 40 years ago, and many technical and methodological advances have been made since.[5] The most widely studied nucleus in cardiac MRS is ^{31}P, with the obtained spectrum being dominated by high-energy phosphate peaks of adenosine triphosphate (ATP) and phosphocreatine (PCr).[6] ^{1}H-MRS is also quite diffuse and allows detection of myocardial fat (triglycerides), lactate, creatine, carnitine, and myoglobin levels.[7]

This review recapitulates the contribution of MRS to current knowledge about cardiac metabolism in the healthy and failing heart, adding general methodological considerations regarding human cardiac MRS. Current applications and potential future developments regarding the use of MRS in HF are also discussed.

METHODOLOGY OF MAGNETIC RESONANCE SPECTROSCOPY

It is beyond the scope of this article to describe the basic principles of MRS in detail, but comprehensive references are available.[8] As already mentioned, MRS techniques can investigate the metabolic processes of tissues by exploiting the magnetic properties of chemical nuclei with an odd number of protons. Cardiac MRS can be applied to characterize myocardial metabolism using the signal produced from a range of those elements to generate a measurable magnetic moment when exposed to a strong external magnetic field. By directing appropriate radiofrequency pulses toward the tissues to be investigated, the magnetic momentum of susceptible nuclei is momentarily modified. At the end of the stimulation, a certain amount of energy is released from the excited nuclei and can be collected as a spectrum.[9]

^{1}H has 1 proton only and is the most abundant element in human tissues, being contained in water molecules and in several other metabolites. Thus, ^{1}H-MRS can produce quite a strong signal.

Additional nuclei with an odd number of protons, such as ^{31}P, ^{13}C, ^{23}Na, and ^{87}Rb, are much less common in the human body, but MRS applications targeting these elements as a potential source of signal have also been developed. However, in the latter case, the production of useful MRS spectra may prove to be more technically difficult.

The first studies on cardiac energetics were conducted in isolated perfused rat hearts in 1977 with ^{31}P-MRS,[10] and in 1984 with ^{1}H-MRS,[11] but it took longer to obtain the same results in human hearts.[12,13] Initial implementations of in vivo MRS were not sensitive enough to warrant routine applicability.[14] However, with the introduction of scanners with high-strength magnetic fields, evolved coils, and optimized radiofrequency pulse designs, sensitivity has been significantly improved.[15] Contemporary hardware requirements for clinical MRS studies include the use of a 1.5 or 3.0 T magnet and, when studying nuclei other than ^{1}H, nucleus-specific coils, and a broadband radiofrequency transmitter. Data acquisition and interpretation are ensured by using MRS acquisition sequences and dedicated postprocessing and data analysis packages.[16]

High magnetic field homogeneity is essential to collect accurate MRS data, and signal quality may be compromised by the effect of motion. To reduce this issue, acquisition of cardiac spectra is performed using cardiac triggering and respiratory gating, and generally takes 15 to 30 minutes.[17] To obtain sufficient signal from the myocardium and avoid signal contamination from blood and epicardial fat, a volume of interest is typically placed in the interventricular septum using appropriate localizer images (**Fig. 1**). The use of standardized and appropriate methodology is crucial to maintain adequate sensitivity and reproducibility of the obtained data.[18]

In cardiology, ^{1}H-MRS and ^{31}P-MRS showed more promise in terms of potential clinical application. ^{1}H-MRS is applied to study cardiac ^{1}H-containing metabolites other than water. In a typical ^{1}H spectrum the water peak at a frequency of 4.7 parts per million (ppm) is prominent, and water suppression techniques need to be implemented to detect myocardial content of nonwater ^{1}H-containing metabolites.[19] Other detectable peaks of ^{1}H-rich metabolites are those of triglycerides (TGs), unsaturated fatty acids (UFAs), creatine (Cr), and choline (see **Fig. 1**). Contributions from lactate is generally superimposed to the triglyceride peaks and cannot be clearly distinguished in the spectra.[20] In vivo, ^{1}H-MRS is more frequently applied to assess TG content, because myocardial lipid overload has been implicated in the pathophysiology of many cardiac conditions, c

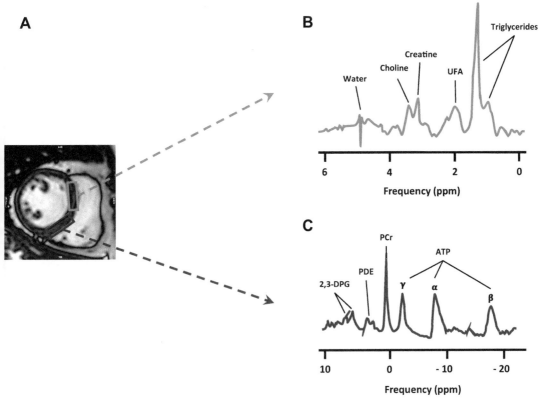

Fig. 1. Examples of cardiac magnetic resonance spectroscopy (MRS) in a healthy individual. (*A*) Mid short-axis localizer image acquired at 1.5 T with voxel selection for ^{1}H-MRS (*blue box*) and ^{31}P-MRS (*red box*); (*B*) typical ^{1}H-MRS spectrum (with water suppression); (*C*) typical ^{31}P-MRS spectrum. 2,3-DGP, 2,3 diphosphoglycerate; ATP, adenosine triphosphate; PDE, phosphodiester; ppm, parts per million; UFA, unsaturated fatty acids.

to measure total myocardial levels of Cr, a key component of the high-energy phosphate system.[7] Myocardial TG level is generally expressed as a ratio of lipid to water, with myocardial TG signals acquired at 1.4 ppm from spectra with water suppression, and water signals acquired at 4.7 ppm from spectra without water suppression.[21]

When observing a typical ^{31}P spectrum from a healthy individual, 6 resonance peaks can be recognized, including 3 ^{31}P atoms (α, β, and γ) of ATP, PCr, phosphodiesters, and 2,3-diphosphoglycerate (see **Fig. 1**). ^{31}P-MRS can provide direct information of myocardial metabolic health, mainly through the assessment of the PCr/ATP ratio, the normal values of which are around 1.5 to 2.0.[22]

CARDIAC ENERGY METABOLISM IN NORMAL AND FAILING HEART

The energy metabolism of the heart requires a continuous supply of nutrients and oxygen to produce ATP, which is the primary carrier of energy in cells. In particular, the healthy heart obtains about 70% of the required energy from long-chain fatty acid oxidation and the rest mostly from cytosolic glycolysis.

In cardiomyocytes, most ATP is synthesized in the mitochondria by oxidative phosphorylation and using energy supplied by fatty acids and glucose (**Fig. 2**).[23] Mitochondrial creatine kinase (CK) catalyzes the transfer of high-energy phosphoryl groups from ATP to Cr, forming PCr and adenosine diphosphate (ADP). Rapidly diffusing PCr connects sites of energy production with sites of energy consumption (CK energy shuttle). At time of high-energy demand, cytosolic CK catalyzes the regeneration of ATP from ADP. The main myocardial ATP-consuming sites are actomyosin ATPase in myofibrils, Ca^{2+}-ATPase in the sarcoplasmic reticulum, and Na^{+}/K^{+}-ATPase in the sarcolemma. At energy-consuming sites, CK isoforms generate ATP from PCr to maintain constant PCr/ATP ratios even during increased workloads.[24]

Proton Myocardial Spectroscopy

In vivo, ^{1}H-MRS has been mainly used to assess the lipid content of the heart (as TGs and UFAs)

Cardiomyocyte

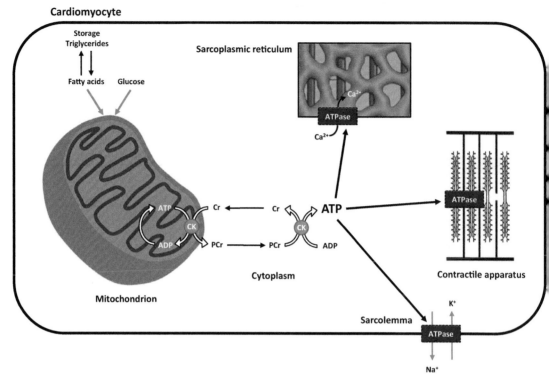

Fig. 2. Schematic representation of the creatine kinase (CK) system in the cardiomyocyte. Energy is constantly transferred under the form of phosphocreatine (PCr) from the mitochondria, where most adenosine triphosphate (ATP) is produced, to the sites of energy consumption. These are mainly represented by the actomyosin ATPase in the contractile apparatus, the Na+/K+-ATPase in the sarcolemma and the sarcoplasmic reticulum Ca2+-ATPase (SERCA), which maintain calcium homeostasis.

and to measure total Cr, a fundamental player in the CK system.

The myocardial lipid pool is highly dynamic, but relatively stable values of TG can be measured in the heart in physiologic conditions (normal TG/water ratio <0.9%).[7] In healthy nonobese individuals, myocardial TG concentration as measured by ^{1}H-MRS seems to be unrelated to gender,[25] but increases with aging (**Fig. 3**).[26,27] Short-term caloric restriction was reported as potentially responsible of increased myocardial TG content,[28,29] whereas endurance physical training reduces the TG pool in the heart.[30]

Epidemiologically, HF is a prevalent condition and, in many cases, myocardial steatosis with TG accumulation could mediate the development of preclinical and clinical ventricular dysfunction.[7] Data obtained in experimental animal models and in human subjects studied by ^{1}H-MRS demonstrated progressive reduction of ventricular function when myocardial TG content increases (**Fig. 4**).[31,32]

It is well known that obesity and type 2 diabetes mellitus are associated with an increased risk of HF, even in absence of ischemic vascular disease.[33,34] Obesity and diabetes are frequently

associated comorbidities, and patients affected by these conditions tend to develop increased left ventricular mass and reduced diastolic and systolic function, as documented by

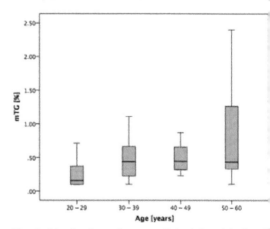

Fig. 3. Distribution of myocardial triglyceride (mTG) content (expressed by percentage relative to unsuppressed water signal) in different age cohorts of healthy volunteers. (*From* Petritsch B, Gassenmaier T, Kunz AS, et al. Age dependency of myocardial triglyceride content: a 3T high-field 1H-MR spectroscopy study. Rofo 2015;187(11):1020; with permission.)

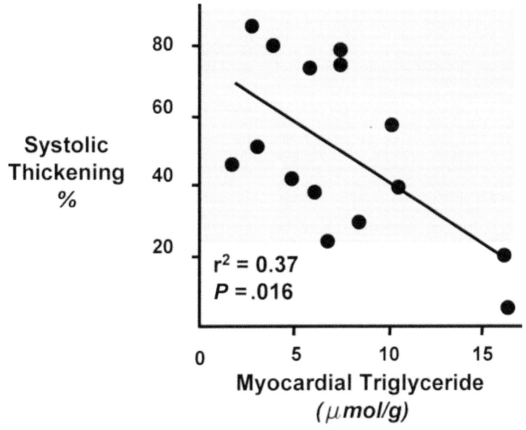

Fig. 4. Myocardial triglyceride content is inversely correlated with the regional systolic function measured as septal thickening. (*From* Szczepaniak LS, Dobbins RL, Metzger GJ, et al. Myocardial triglycerides and systolic function in humans: in vivo evaluation by localized proton spectroscopy and cardiac imaging. Magn Reson Med 2003;49(3):422; with permission.)

echocardiography and MRI.[35,36] Body mass index (BMI) is a major determinant of myocardial TG content, and the TG/water ratio increases linearly with BMI.[37] Consequently, myocardial fat content is markedly increased in obese compared with nonobese individuals.[38] TG accumulation as measured by ^{1}H-MRS also occurs in patients with diabetes.[39]

In the heart, excess lipid may be stored as TGs in the cytoplasm, but also shunted into nonoxidative pathways that disrupt normal cellular signaling, ultimately leading to cell damage (lipotoxicity).[40] In patients with uncomplicated diabetes, Rijzewijk and colleagues[41] reported increased myocardial TG content and an association with impaired diastolic ventricular function independently of age and BMI. Interestingly, whereas in healthy controls a very low calorie diet may produce a significant increase in myocardial TG content and associated diastolic dysfunction,[29] in obese patients with diabetes an increased basal myocardial TG pool may be

corrected with dietary restriction, with a matching improvement in diastolic ventricular function.[42] These and other studies demonstrated that myocardial TG stores are flexible and may represent a potential target for therapeutic intervention.

Cardiac adiposity, with ectopic fat accumulation within the heart and around it (epicardial and pericardial fat) has an established importance in development of cardiovascular diseases.[43] Using ^{1}H-MRS and cardiac MRI in patients with HF owing to dilated cardiomyopathy, Granér and colleagues[44] observed a decreased myocardial TG content and increased epicardial/pericardial fat deposition as an expression of severe derangement of fat metabolism. Unfortunately, limited and conflicting data have been reported regarding changes in lipid metabolism observed in HF and, so far, attempts to identify a unique pattern of modification were unproductive.[45] In fact, Nakae and colleagues[43] failed to demonstrate significant differences in myocardial TG content between patients with dilated cardiomyopathy and controls. These discordant results could be explained by considering myocardial TG as a cause-specific marker rather than expression of the severity of the disease in HF, but appropriate data still need to be produced.

In the myocardium, ^{1}H-MRS can also be applied to measure total Cr (composed of free Cr and PCr), and this can be obtained with sufficient sensitivity when the CrEST (chemical exchange saturation transfer) technique is implemented.[46] Myocardial Cr levels are consistently reduced in the failing heart, regardless of cause, and correlate with the function of the left ventricle (LV).[47,48] This was demonstrated in studies including small samples of patients and needs to be confirmed in larger populations. Of interest, in patients with HF the decrease in total Cr seems to precede the ATP decline, as observed in the more advanced stages of the disease, supporting the energy-starvation hypothesis of the failing heart as developed by some investigators.[24,49]

Phosphorus Myocardial Spectroscopy

After extensive initial experimental experiences (ex vivo and in situ open chest animal models),[10,50] ^{31}P-MRS finally developed into a unique noninvasive technique that allows in vivo detection of ^{31}P-containing metabolites involved in energy metabolism of the heart.[51]

In cardiomyocytes, the CK system is always in a near-equilibrium state and the PCr/ATP ratio is generally used as an index of cardiac energy status. Bioenergetics impairment in the failing heart is reflected by a decrease in cardiac ATP, PCr, and PCr/ATP ratio.[52,53] In 1997, Neubauer and colleagues[54] found the PCr/ATP ratio to be a better prognostic marker than some traditional indices of functional status, such as New York Heart Association Class and LV ejection fraction in patients with dilated cardiomyopathy of ischemic or idiopathic origin (**Fig. 5**). Unfortunately, that experience remained isolated, with later studies failing to observe reduced PCr/ATP ratios in hearts of patients with dilated cardiomyopathy.[51]

Additional lines of research suggested the possibility that cardiac PCr/ATP ratio, as measured by ^{31}P-MRS, could correlate with HF severity. In patients with HF with reduced ejection fraction (HFrEF), a significant correlation was observed between cardiac PCr/ATP ratio and ejection fraction.[55] However, in about half of patients with HF symptoms, this clinical syndrome is not associated with significantly reduced LV ejection fraction. HF with preserved ejection fraction (HFpEF) is an under-investigated condition, in which the search for useful prognostic markers is even more desirable.[56] Ventricular systole and diastole are both active processes that use ATP. Thus, in HFpEF, excessive energy is consumed to maintain the abnormally increased diastolic tension. The myocardial PCr/ATP ratio is reduced in HFrEF and is associated with diastolic dysfunction.[57,58]

Obesity and diabetes have been associated with diastolic dysfunction and with predisposition to develop HF.[59] In a study conducted using cardiac MRI and ^{31}P-MRS in obese patients, Rider and colleagues[60] found the cardiac PCr/ATP ratio to be the only independent predictor of diastolic dysfunction on multivariable analysis, suggesting myocardial energetics as a key player in the development of diastolic dysfunction in obesity. On the contrary, weight loss in obese patients was associated to improved cardiac PCr/ATP and diastolic function.[61]

The altered myocardial energetic status as measured by cardiac ^{31}P-MRS has been proposed as an imaging biomarker to assess HF severity, but also to monitor clinical response to therapy. In particular, the cardiac PCr/ATP ratio shows improvement during clinical recompensation with standard HF treatment.[22] In patients with diabetes, data regarding the link between altered myocardial bioenergetics and diastolic dysfunction were more conflicting.[51] Cardiac PCr/ATP ratio and LV function may not be correlated in many patients with preclinical or overt HF, because many other processes may regulate the development of myocardial dysfunction, including fibrosis, oxidative stress, and altered calcium homeostasis.[62]

Some preclinical studies and small clinical trials suggested the possibility to use polyphenols (including resveratrol and epicatechin naturally found in foods such as dark chocolate, dark tea, or red wine to stimulate mitochondrial biogenesis.[63,64] Perhexiline is an inhibitor of mitochondrial carnitine palmitoyltransferase-1 used as an antianginal agent and proposed for patients with HF based on the demonstration of favorable effects on LV ejection fraction and functional class.[65] In a placebo-controlled study involving patients with nonischemic HF, perhexiline short-term therapy was associated with a 30% increase in myocardial PCr/ATP ratio versus a 3% decrease with placebo, with concomitant improvement in functional class (**Fig. 6**).[66]

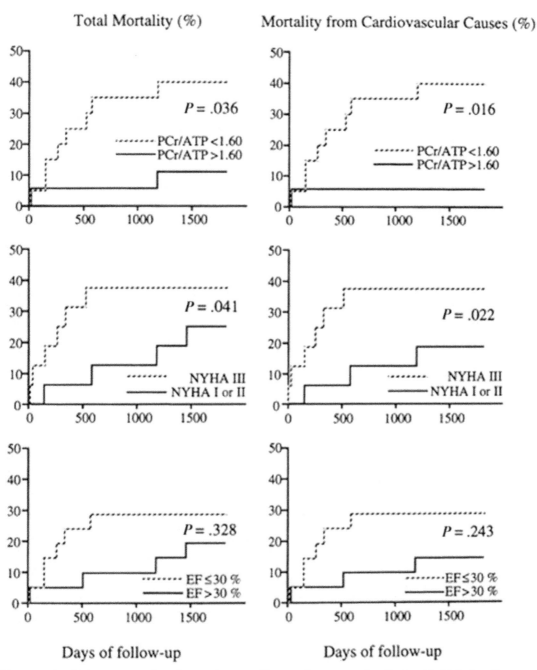

Fig. 5. Kaplan-Meier analyses of cardiovascular mortality rates for groups of patients with dilated cardiomyopathy split by phosphocreatine/adenosine triphosphate (PCr/ATP) ratio, New York Heart Association class, or left ventricular ejection fraction (EF). PCr/ATP ratio is identified as a sensitive predictor of cardiovascular mortality. (*From* Neubauer S, Horn M, Cramer M, et al. Myocardial phosphocreatine-to-ATP ratio is a predictor of mortality in patients with dilated cardiomyopathy. Circulation 1997;96(7):2190–6; with permission.)

PITFALLS

With cardiac MRS, fundamental technical limitations still restrain the full exploitation of its clinical potential. As mentioned earlier, this technique interrogates nonproton nuclei and nonwater ^{1}H-containing metabolites, which are present in concentrations several orders of magnitude lower than ^{1}H in water molecules. As a direct consequence, cardiac MRS signals are about

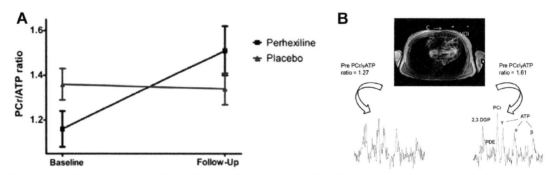

Fig. 6. Favorable therapeutic effects of perhexiline on myocardial efficiency in heart failure. (*A*) Effects of perhexiline over 1 month in patients with symptomatic, nonischemic dilated cardiomyopathy on cardiac phosphocreatine/adenosine triphosphate (PCr/ATP) ratio. (*B*) Example of ^{31}P-MRS before and after treatment with perhexiline, with significant increase in PCr/ATP ratio. (*From* Beadle RM, Williams LK, Kuehl M, et al. Improvement in cardiac energetics by perhexiline in heart failure due to dilated cardiomyopathy. JACC Heart Fail 2015;3(3):208 with permission.)

100 times weaker than those of clinical MRI, requiring many signal averages and, thus, longer scanning times.[67] Predictably, for cardiac MRS, this translates into poor spatial (larger voxel sizes) and limited temporal resolution. Furthermore, the use of large voxels may incur the risk of including contamination from noncardiac signal sources, thus resulting in high measurement variability.[7] When studying the moving heart, the acquired signal intensity may be further reduced because of the effects of the same strategies implemented to limit the negative impact of cardiac and respiratory motion on data quality.[4] The effects of motion may also hamper the efficiency of water suppression techniques applied to remove the dominant water signal. Finally, postprocessing for cardiac MRS may be particularly demanding and needs full understanding of both cardiac physiopathology and technical challenges.

During the last decades, as a result of the lack of expertise and of advanced hardware and software tools, only few centers have been actively involved in research activities involving cardiac MRS. Demonstration of potential clinical use with cardiac MRS will certainly depend on substantial technical developments (see the following paragraph) and use of higher magnetic field strengths (which are still scantily available). Predictably, a wide diffusion of cardiac MRS will not be obtained in the short term.[68]

FUTURE PERSPECTIVES

Implementation of MRS in clinical practice will only become a reality if MRS signals can be augmented substantially. One straightforward way to do so is based on the implementation of high-field and ultra-high-field systems for clinical MRS. Cardiac MRS methodology at 3 T has been recently standardized, and modern clinical systems provide data with high intrasession and intersession reproducibility.[69] The improved chemical shift resolution and signal-to-noise ratio of cardiac ^{1}H-MRS with high-field scanners allowed new applications such as the discrimination between fatty acids and UFA deposition in the myocardium.[45] The use of ultra-high magnetic field (7 T) scanners might provide further benefits in terms of sensitivity and resolution, with the potential possibility to investigate cardiac energetic metabolism in more detail, extending the options available for clinical research (**Fig. 7**).[53,70] It could even offer the chance of detecting ventricular energetic anomalies at a regional level and, with improved temporal resolution, real-time assessment of the temporal changes in regional processes will probably become a reality. Some investigators predict that 7 T will developed as the hardware setting of choice for cardiac MRS.[71] Additional technical implementations, such as the use of advanced shimming algorithms, multichannel detection coils, hyperpolarized nuclei, and Dixon MRI promise further improvement in clinical applicability for noninvasive evaluation of cardiac metabolism.[72]

Within the various noninvasive readouts of cardiac energy status provided by ^{31}P-MRS, the PCr/ATP ratio is the easiest to obtain. However, the absolute concentrations of PCr and ATP would be more sensitive markers of cardiac bioenergetics status and changes, because the PCr/ATP ratio is obviously insensitive to similar variations in both parameters. Implementation of quantitative measurements of high-energy ^{31}P peaks from cardiac MRS spectra is challenging: measurements may be affected by various technical aspects (eg, magnetic field homogeneity, radiofrequency coils sensitivity profile); reference values for

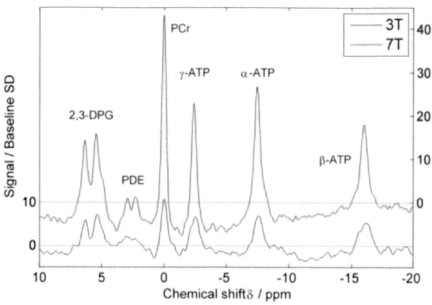

Fig. 7. Comparison of 3T versus 7T spectra obtained in the same individual with ^{31}P-MRS. An increased signal-to-noise ratio (SNR) at 7 T is clearly evident. (*From* Rodgers CT, Clarke WT, Snyder C, et al. Human cardiac 31P magnetic resonance spectroscopy at 7 Tesla. Magn Reson Med 2014;72(2):311; with permission.)

absolute concentrations are needed.[51] Initial experiences reported the implementation of absolute ^{31}P quantification in humans,[73] observing a concomitant (but differential) reduction of both PCr and ATP in patients with HF due to dilated cardiomyopathy.[74]

SUMMARY

Although MRI predominantly relies on ^{1}H nuclei in water as the main signal source, MRS allows the study of many other nuclei with odd numbers of protons, including ^{31}P, ^{13}C, [23]Na, [87]Rb, and [1]H (in metabolites other than water). MRS already has solid clinical application in neuroimaging and it is rapidly finding a place in prostate and breast imaging. Cardiac MRS certainly has considerable potential and is the only available method for the noninvasive assessment of cardiac metabolism without external radioactive tracers. However, even though initial in vivo studies using MRS to assess cardiac pathology were reported several decades ago, this technique is still struggling to find a place in clinical cardiology.

In recent years, considerable technical and methodological developments have certainly improved clinical applicability of MRS.[75] Recently, dedicated scientific statements have been reported in recognition of the growing relevance of the methods proposed for the assessment of cardiac metabolism and of the potential to improve

the function of the failing heart by targeting abnormalities in cardiac energy metabolism.[67,76] However, cardiac MRS remains a technically complex method and, up to now, requires increased expertise and dedicated setup. The acquisition of solid data with cardiac MRS is still challenging because of some intrinsic physical limitations: nonproton nuclei have a much lower signal sensitivity than ^{1}H and, at the same time, metabolites interrogated with MRS are present in concentrations several orders of magnitude lower than those of ^{1}H nuclei in water.[67]

The failing heart is the perfect setting to challenge the presumptive ability of MRS to recognize in vivo anomalies in cardiac bioenergetics. The heart requires a constant supply of balanced nutrients (primarily glucose and lipids) to produce the required amount of ATP, which is the principal source of energy for most cellular functions.[72] ^{1}H-MRS has been mainly used in defining the variations in cardiac TG content, trying to recognize the prodromes to cell damage from lipid excess (lipotoxicity). So far, however, any attempt to recognize a typical pattern of modification in lipid metabolism with cardiac ^{1}H-MRS in patients with HF has been unproductive.[45] Instead, more convincing data confirmed that the failing heart is energy starved. Using ^{31}P-MRS in HF, a large number of studies found a reduced PCr/ATP ratio to be a reliable marker of impaired bioenergetics, correlating with a hampered cardiac functional status.[49] Also, cardiac MRS is a promising new

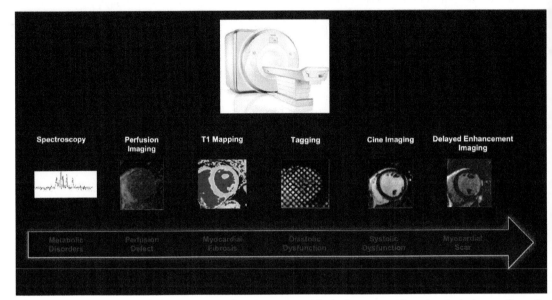

Fig. 8. Cardiac MRI in heart failure. A comprehensive protocol including several imaging techniques allows the assessment of abnormalities in cardiac metabolism, ventricular tissue characteristics, myocardial perfusion, and function involving the failing heart.

tool to study the effects of nutritional and pharmacologic interventions on myocardial metabolism in relation to heart function, particularly in obese patients with diabetes.[76,77] The favorable clinical results obtained with some novel drugs recently introduced in HF treatment schemes, including angiotensin receptor blocker-neprilysin inhibitor and sodium glucose cotransporter 2 inhibitors, have been at least partly attributed to their effects on cardiac metabolism.[78]

Impaired cellular energy production and transfer have been confirmed as key components of the metabolic processes involved in the development and clinical course of HFrEF and HEFpEF.[79] Within the wide range of conditions potentially responsible for HF symptoms, there is still debate about the existence of distinct disorders such as diabetic cardiomyopathy and obesity cardiomyopathy.[80,81] However, the development of these clinical conditions cannot be completely explained by traditional risk factors, and a deeper evaluation of associated myocardial metabolic abnormalities obtained with MRS could be particularly helpful in shedding new light on the underlying mechanisms.

Cardiac MRI already has a central role in the management of HF.[82] In clinical practice, comprehensive MRI protocols applied to the study of patients with HF allow a full characterization of the structural and functional abnormalities observed in this condition (**Fig. 8**).[83] In the future, inclusion of noninvasive assessment of cardiac bioenergetics using MRS could allow a better definition

of the most appropriate diagnostic and therapeutic strategies for each patient with HF.

REFERENCES

1. Lesyuk W, Kriza C, Kolominsky-Rabas P. Cost-of-illness studies in heart failure: a systematic review 2004-2016. BMC Cardiovasc Disord 2018 18:74.
2. Francis GS. Pathophysiology of chronic heart failure Am J Med 2001;110(Suppl 7A):37S–46S.
3. Faghihi R, Zeinali-Rafsanjani B, Mosleh-Shirazi M-A et al. Magnetic resonance spectroscopy and its clinical applications: a review. J Med Imaging Radia Sci 2017;48:233–53.
4. Qureshi WT, Nasir UB. Principals and clinical applications of magnetic resonance cardiac spectroscopy in heart failure. Heart Fail Rev 2017;22:491–9
5. Garlick PB, Radda GK, Seeley PJ. Phosphorus NMR studies on perfused heart. Biochem Biophys Res Commun 1977;74:1256–62.
6. Ingwall JS, Kramer MF, Fifer MA, et al. The creatine kinase system in normal and diseased human myocardium. N Engl J Med 1985;313:1050–4.
7. Faller KME, Lygate CA, Neubauer S, et al. (1)H-MR spectroscopy for analysis of cardiac lipid and creatine metabolism. Heart Fail Rev 2013;18:657–68.
8. van der Graaf M. In vivo magnetic resonance spectroscopy: basic methodology and clinical applications. Eur Biophys J 2010;39:527–40.
9. Dellegrottaglie S, Rajagopalan S. Fundamental principles of MR imaging. In: Mukherjee D Rajagopalan S, editors. CT and MR angiography of

the peripheral circulation. Essex (England): CRC Press; 2007. p. 147–61.

10. Jacobus WE, Taylor GJ, Hollis DP, et al. Phosphorus nuclear magnetic resonance of perfused working rat hearts. Nature 1977;265:756–8.

11. Ugurbil K, Petein M, Maidan R, et al. High resolution proton NMR studies of perfused rat hearts. FEBS Lett 1984;167:73–8.

12. Bottomley PA. Noninvasive study of high-energy phosphate metabolism in human heart by depth-resolved 31P NMR spectroscopy. Science 1985;229:769–72.

13. den Hollander JA, Evanochko WT, Pohost GM. Observation of cardiac lipids in humans by localized 1H magnetic resonance spectroscopic imaging. Magn Reson Med 1994;32:175–80.

14. Fossel ET, Morgan HE, Ingwall JS. Measurement of changes in high-energy phosphates in the cardiac cycle using gated 31P nuclear magnetic renonance. Proc Natl Acad Sci U S A 1980;77:3654–8.

15. Löffler R, Sauter R, Kolem H, et al. Localized spectroscopy from anatomically matched compartments: improved sensitivity and localization for cardiac 31P MRS in humans. J Magn Reson 1998;134:287–99.

16. Naressi A, Couturier C, Castang I, et al. Java-based graphical user interface for MRUI, a software package for quantitation of in vivo/medical magnetic resonance spectroscopy signals. Comput Biol Med 2001;31:269–86.

17. Gastl M, Peereboom SM, Fuetterer M, et al. Cardiac-versus diaphragm-based respiratory navigation for proton spectroscopy of the heart. MAGMA 2019; 32:259–68.

18. Reingold JS, McGavock JM, Kaka S, et al. Determination of triglyceride in the human myocardium by magnetic resonance spectroscopy: reproducibility and sensitivity of the method. Am J Physiol Endocrinol Metab 2005;289:E935–9.

19. Haase A, Frahm J, Hänicke W, et al. 1H NMR chemical shift selective (CHESS) imaging. Phys Med Biol 1985;30:341–4.

20. Walecki J, Michalak MJ, Michalak E, et al. Usefulness of 1H MR spectroscopy in the evaluation of myocardial metabolism in patients with dilated idiopathic cardiomyopathy: pilot study. Acad Radiol 2003;10:1187–92.

21. Felblinger J, Jung B, Slotboom J, et al. Methods and reproducibility of cardiac/respiratory double-triggered (1)H-MR spectroscopy of the human heart. Magn Reson Med 1999;42:903–10.

22. Neubauer S, Krahe T, Schindler R, et al. 31P magnetic resonance spectroscopy in dilated cardiomyopathy and coronary artery disease. Altered cardiac high-energy phosphate metabolism in heart failure. Circulation 1992;86:1810–8.

23. Guzun R, Timohhina N, Tepp K, et al. Systems bioenergetics of creatine kinase networks: physiological roles of creatine and phosphocreatine in regulation of cardiac cell function. Amino Acids 2011;40:1333–48.

24. Ingwall JS, Weiss RG. Is the failing heart energy starved? On using chemical energy to support cardiac function. Circ Res 2004;95:135–45.

25. Petritsch B, Köstler H, Gassenmaier T, et al. An investigation into potential gender-specific differences in myocardial triglyceride content assessed by 1H-magnetic resonance spectroscopy at 3Tesla. J Int Med Res 2016;44:585–91.

26. van der Meer RW, Rijzewijk LJ, Diamant M, et al. The ageing male heart: myocardial triglyceride content as independent predictor of diastolic function. Eur Heart J 2008;29:1516–22.

27. Petritsch B, Gassenmaier T, Kunz AS, et al. Age dependency of myocardial triglyceride content: a 3T high-field 1H-MR spectroscopy study. ROFO Fortschr Geb Rontgenstr Nuklearmed 2015;187:1016–21.

28. Hammer S, van der Meer RW, Lamb HJ, et al. Progressive caloric restriction induces dose-dependent changes in myocardial triglyceride content and diastolic function in healthy men. J Clin Endocrinol Metab 2008;93:497–503.

29. van der Meer RW, Hammer S, Smit JWA, et al. Short-term caloric restriction induces accumulation of myocardial triglycerides and decreases left ventricular diastolic function in healthy subjects. Diabetes 2007;56:2849–53.

30. Sai E, Shimada K, Yokoyama T, et al. Association between myocardial triglyceride content and cardiac function in healthy subjects and endurance athletes. PLoS One 2013;8:e61604.

31. Hankiewicz JH, Banke NH, Farjah M, et al. Early impairment of transmural principal strains in the left ventricular wall after short-term, high-fat feeding of mice predisposed to cardiac steatosis. Circ Cardiovasc Imaging 2010;3:710–7.

32. Szczepaniak LS, Dobbins RL, Metzger GJ, et al. Myocardial triglycerides and systolic function in humans: in vivo evaluation by localized proton spectroscopy and cardiac imaging. Magn Reson Med 2003;49:417–23.

33. Aune D, Sen A, Norat T, et al. Body mass index, abdominal fatness, and heart failure incidence and mortality: a systematic review and dose-response meta-analysis of prospective studies. Circulation 2016;133:639–49.

34. Zhou L, Deng W, Zhou L, et al. Prevalence, incidence and risk factors of chronic heart failure in the type 2 diabetic population: systematic review. Curr Diabetes Rev 2009;5:171–84.

35. Lauer MS, Anderson KM, Kannel WB, et al. The impact of obesity on left ventricular mass and geometry. The Framingham Heart Study. JAMA 1991;266: 231–6.

36. Shah RV, Abbasi SA, Heydari B, et al. Insulin resistance, subclinical left ventricular remodeling, and the

obesity paradox: MESA (Multi-Ethnic Study of Atherosclerosis). J Am Coll Cardiol 2013;61:1698–706.

37. Rial B, Robson MD, Neubauer S, et al. Rapid quantification of myocardial lipid content in humans using single breath-hold 1H MRS at 3 Tesla. Magn Reson Med 2011;66:619–24.

38. Kankaanpää M, Lehto H-R, Pärkkä JP, et al. Myocardial triglyceride content and epicardial fat mass in human obesity: relationship to left ventricular function and serum free fatty acid levels. J Clin Endocrinol Metab 2006;91:4689–95.

39. McGavock JM, Lingvay I, Zib I, et al. Cardiac steatosis in diabetes mellitus: a 1H-magnetic resonance spectroscopy study. Circulation 2007;116:1170–5.

40. Wende AR, Abel ED. Lipotoxicity in the heart. Biochim Biophys Acta 2010;1801:311–9.

41. Rijzewijk LJ, van der Meer RW, Lamb HJ, et al. Altered myocardial substrate metabolism and decreased diastolic function in nonischemic human diabetic cardiomyopathy: studies with cardiac positron emission tomography and magnetic resonance imaging. J Am Coll Cardiol 2009;54:1524–32.

42. Hammer S, Snel M, Lamb HJ, et al. Prolonged caloric restriction in obese patients with type 2 diabetes mellitus decreases myocardial triglyceride content and improves myocardial function. J Am Coll Cardiol 2008;52:1006–12.

43. Nakae I, Mitsunami K, Yoshino T, et al. Clinical features of myocardial triglyceride in different types of cardiomyopathy assessed by proton magnetic resonance spectroscopy: comparison with myocardial creatine. J Card Fail 2010;16:812–22.

44. Granér M, Pentikäinen MO, Nyman K, et al. Cardiac steatosis in patients with dilated cardiomyopathy. Heart 2014;100:1107–12.

45. Liao P-A, Lin G, Tsai S-Y, et al. Myocardial triglyceride content at 3 T cardiovascular magnetic resonance and left ventricular systolic function: a cross-sectional study in patients hospitalized with acute heart failure. J Cardiovasc Magn Reson 2016;18:9.

46. Haris M, Singh A, Cai K, et al. A technique for in vivo mapping of myocardial creatine kinase metabolism. Nat Med 2014;20:209–14.

47. Lygate CA, Fischer A, Sebag-Montefiore L, et al. The creatine kinase energy transport system in the failing mouse heart. J Mol Cell Cardiol 2007;42:1129–36.

48. Nakae I, Mitsunami K, Omura T, et al. Proton magnetic resonance spectroscopy can detect creatine depletion associated with the progression of heart failure in cardiomyopathy. J Am Coll Cardiol 2003;42:1587–93.

49. Neubauer S. The failing heart – an engine out of fuel. N Engl J Med 2007;356:1140–51.

50. Grove TH, Ackerman JJ, Radda GK, et al. Analysis of rat heart in vivo by phosphorus nuclear magnetic resonance. Proc Natl Acad Sci U S A 1980;77:299–302.

51. Abdurrachim D, Prompers JJ. Evaluation of cardiac energetics by non-invasive 31P magnetic resonance spectroscopy. Biochim Biophys Acta Mol Basis Dis 2018;1864:1939–48.

52. Hardy CJ, Weiss RG, Bottomley PA, et al. Altered myocardial high-energy phosphate metabolites in patients with dilated cardiomyopathy. Am Heart J 1991;122:795–801.

53. Stoll VM, Clarke WT, Levelt E, et al. Dilated cardiomyopathy: phosphorus 31 MR spectroscopy at 7 T. Radiology 2016;281:409–17.

54. Neubauer S, Horn M, Cramer M, et al. Myocardial phosphocreatine-to-ATP ratio is a predictor of mortality in patients with dilated cardiomyopathy. Circulation 1997;96:2190–6.

55. Hansch A, Rzanny R, Heyne J-P, et al. Noninvasive measurements of cardiac high-energy phosphate metabolites in dilated cardiomyopathy by using 31P spectroscopic chemical shift imaging. Eur Radiol 2005;15:319–23.

56. Yancy CW, Jessup M, Bozkurt B, et al. 2017 ACC/AHA/HFSA focused update of the 2013 ACCF/AHA guideline for the management of heart failure: A Report of the American College of Cardiology/American Heart Association Task Force on Clinical Practice Guidelines and the Heart Failure Society of America. Circulation 2017;136:e137–61.

57. Lamb HJ, Beyerbacht HP, van der Laarse A, et al. Diastolic dysfunction in hypertensive heart disease is associated with altered myocardial metabolism. Circulation 1999;99:2261–7.

58. Phan TT, Abozguia K, Nallur Shivu G, et al. Heart failure with preserved ejection fraction is characterized by dynamic impairment of active relaxation and contraction of the left ventricle on exercise and associated with myocardial energy deficiency. J Am Coll Cardiol 2009;54:402–9.

59. Peterson LR, Waggoner AD, Schechtman KB, et al. Alterations in left ventricular structure and function in young healthy obese women: assessment by echocardiography and tissue Doppler imaging. J Am Coll Cardiol 2004;43:1399–404.

60. Rider OJ, Francis JM, Ali MK, et al. Effects of catecholamine stress on diastolic function and myocardial energetics in obesity. Circulation 2012;125:1511–9.

61. Rider OJ, Francis JM, Tyler D, et al. Effects of weight loss on myocardial energetics and diastolic function in obesity. Int J Cardiovasc Imaging 2013;29:1043–50.

62. Abdurrachim D, Ciapaite J, Wessels B, et al. Cardiac diastolic dysfunction in high-fat diet fed mice is associated with lipotoxicity without impairment of cardiac energetics in vivo. Biochim Biophys Acta 2014;1842:1525–37.

63. Sung MM, Dyck JRB. Therapeutic potential of resveratrol in heart failure. Ann N Y Acad Sci 2015; 1348:32–45.

64. Ramirez-Sanchez I, Taub PR, Ciaraldi TP, et al. (-)-Epicatechin rich cocoa mediated modulation of oxidative stress regulators in skeletal muscle of heart failure and type 2 diabetes patients. Int J Cardiol 2013;168:3982–90.

65. George CH, Mitchell AN, Preece R, et al. Pleiotropic mechanisms of action of perhexiline in heart failure. Expert Opin Ther Pat 2016;26:1049–59.

66. Beadle RM, Williams LK, Kuehl M, et al. Improvement in cardiac energetics by perhexiline in heart failure due to dilated cardiomyopathy. JACC Heart Fail 2015;3:202–11.

67. Taegtmeyer H, Young ME, Lopaschuk GD, et al. American Heart Association Council on Basic Cardiovascular Sciences. Assessing cardiac metabolism: a scientific statement from the American Heart Association. Circ Res 2016;118: 1659–701.

68. Hudsmith LE, Neubauer S. Magnetic resonance spectroscopy in myocardial disease. JACC Cardiovasc Imaging 2009;2:87–96.

69. de Heer P, Bizino MB, Lamb HJ, et al. Parameter optimization for reproducible cardiac 1 H-MR spectroscopy at 3 Tesla. J Magn Reson Imaging 2016;44: 1151–8.

70. Rodgers CT, Clarke WT, Snyder C, et al. Human cardiac 31P magnetic resonance spectroscopy at 7 Tesla. Magn Reson Med 2014;72:304–15.

71. Valkovič L, Dragonu I, Almujayyaz S, et al. Using a whole-body 31P birdcage transmit coil and 16-element receive array for human cardiac metabolic imaging at 7T. PLoS One 2017;12: e0187153.

72. van Ewijk PA, Schrauwen-Hinderling VB, Bekkers SCAM, et al. MRS: a noninvasive window into cardiac metabolism. NMR Biomed 2015;28: 747–66.

73. Meininger M, Landschütz W, Beer M, et al. Concentrations of human cardiac phosphorus metabolites determined by SLOOP 31P NMR spectroscopy. Magn Reson Med 1999;41:657–63.

74. Beer M, Seyfarth T, Sandstede J, et al. Absolute concentrations of high-energy phosphate metabolites in normal, hypertrophied, and failing human myocardium measured noninvasively with (31)P-SLOOP magnetic resonance spectroscopy. J Am Coll Cardiol 2002;40:1267–74.

75. Scally C, Rudd A, Mezincescu A, et al. Persistent long-term structural, functional, and metabolic changes after stress-induced (Takotsubo) cardiomyopathy. Circulation 2018;137:1039–48.

76. Brown DA, Perry JB, Allen ME, et al. Expert consensus document: mitochondrial function as a therapeutic target in heart failure. Nat Rev Cardiol 2017;14:238–50.

77. Lamb HJ, Smit JW, van der Meer RW, et al. Metabolic MRI of myocardial and hepatic triglyceride content in response to nutritional interventions. Curr Opin Clin Nutr Metab Care 2008;11:573–9.

78. Birkenfeld AL, Jordan J, Dworak M, et al. Myocardial metabolism in heart failure: purinergic signalling and other metabolic concepts. Pharmacol Ther 2019; 194:132–44.

79. Lewis GA, Schelbert EB, Williams SG, et al. Biological phenotypes of heart failure with preserved ejection fraction. J Am Coll Cardiol 2017;70:2186–200.

80. Schilling JD, Mann DL. Diabetic cardiomyopathy: bench to bedside. Heart Fail Clin 2012;8:619–31.

81. Wong C, Marwick TH. Obesity cardiomyopathy: pathogenesis and pathophysiology. Nat Clin Pract Cardiovasc Med 2007;4:436–43.

82. Patel MR, White RD, Abbara S, et al. American College of Radiology Appropriateness Criteria Committee, American College of Cardiology Foundation Appropriate Use Criteria Task Force. 2013 ACCF/ ACR/ASE/ASNC/SCCT/SCMR appropriate utilization of cardiovascular imaging in heart failure: a joint report of the American College of Radiology Appropriateness Criteria Committee and the American College of Cardiology Foundation Appropriate Use Criteria Task Force. J Am Coll Cardiol 2013;61: 2207–31.

83. Yoneyama K, Kitanaka Y, Tanaka O, et al. Cardiovascular magnetic resonance imaging in heart failure. Expert Rev Cardiovasc Ther 2018;16:237–48.

Moving?

Make sure your subscription moves with you!

To notify us of your new address, find your **Clinics Account Number** (located on your mailing label above your name), and contact customer service at:

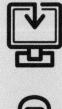

Email: journalscustomerservice-usa@elsevier.com

800-654-2452 (subscribers in the U.S. & Canada)
314-447-8871 (subscribers outside of the U.S. & Canada)

Fax number: 314-447-8029

Elsevier Health Sciences Division
Subscription Customer Service
3251 Riverport Lane
Maryland Heights, MO 63043

*To ensure uninterrupted delivery of your subscription, please notify us at least 4 weeks in advance of move.

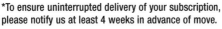